What others are say
Childbirth Manual:

"This is the finest reference guide to homeopathic care for pregnancy, birth, and the newborn I have read. The philosophy of birth being a healthful process in a family's life is echoed throughout the book. Ms. Idarius continues the legacy of midwifery; to be "with women," listening with open heart and mind. This valuable resource manual gives me the guidance and confidence to broaden my use of homeopathic remedies in my midwifery practice. Thank you for such an eloquent, gentle, and thorough compendium of homeopathy for the childbearing woman and her newborn."

> —Laura Mann, C.N.M., F.N.P., M.S., faculty at the Frontier School of Midwifery and Family Nursing, course coordinator of Promoting Health and Wellness, Welcoming Home Nurse-Midwifery Service

"Ms. Idarius has done a great service with this fine manual. The homeopathic information is beautifully presented — in a highly lucid fashion. It is clear that she is not only speaking from many years of experience with the subject, but even more valuable, that she brings to it a sensitivity arising out of a deep love of this work. Bravo!"

> —Ana Chavarria de Shore, P.A.-C., Homeopath/Women's Health

"This book is indispensable to the homeopathic management of the birthing experience."

> —Greg Bedayn, R.S.Hom.(N.A.), C.C.H., editor of *The American Homeopath*

The Homeopathic Childbirth Manual

A practical guide for labor, birth, and the immediate postpartum period

Betty Idarius, L.M., C.Hom.

Published by:

Idarius Press
P.O. Box 388
Talmage, CA 95481
(707) 463-3739
E-mail: bidarius@saber.net
Website: www.saber.net/~bidarius

ISBN 0-9649304-9-8

Cover design by David Paulley of Ram Graphics,
Oakland, California

Printed in the United States of America on
acid-free recycled paper

2 3 4 5 6 — 03 02 01 00 99

Note to the reader: This book has a large inner margin to
allow for spiral binding.

For ordering information refer to the book order form on
the back page.

*Dedicated to
midwives everywhere
and the women they serve
who continue to keep the
wisdom of birth alive*

Acknowledgements

My respect and gratitude go to the modern day homeopaths who have shared their wisdom and experience of using homeopathy during childbirth. These include Ananda Zaren, Dr. Richard Moscowitz, Miranda Castro, Jana Shiloh, Pat Kramer, and Patty Brennan. Their work has served as the foundation for my knowledge in this area.

A special appreciation goes to the many women, and their families, who allowed me to be an intimate part of their lives during pregnancy, birth, and the post-partum period.

The birth of this book was possible only through the support and hard work of many people. I want to thank all those who generously gave of their time to read the original manuscript and offered their valuable suggestions for its improvement.

Any editorial style that this book possesses is due to the patience and attention to detail of Marcia Peterson. Though I wanted to throw the manuscript off the top of a very high mountain after receiving her many original comments, I am glad we both stayed with it.

My gratitude goes to Jack Travis for his many hours of technical support during the preparation of this manuscript, as well as for his friendship.

I am also grateful to Greg Bedayn for his encouragement and assistance in the final stages of preparing this book for press, and to David Paulley for masterfully and patiently designing the book's cover.

My appreciation goes to the Pacific Academy of

Homeopathic Medicine. In particular, I am grateful to Lynn Amara and Jo Daly for their inspiration and enduring commitment to teaching the art and science of homeopathy.

Thanks also to M.J. Hanafin, C.N.M. and homeopath, for sharing with me her insights and experience with the remedy *Crotalus horridus*.

Words can not express the gratitude I feel for my husband, Eric, without whom many of my heart's dreams, including this book, would never have been realized. I am truly blessed to have such a loving partner who sees into my soul and encourages my unfoldment, all with so much tenderness.

Thank you also to my sweet Benjamin, for being born and letting me be his mommie; and for his understanding when I spent so much time at school and with my computer.

Most of all my heart goes to my spiritual teacher, who has brought Divine purpose and direction into my life.

Contents

Preface

Childbirth is a special time in a woman's life, a time of evolution when she blossoms into motherhood, and the family is born. It is the second gateway of initiation towards embodying her inherent female wisdom (the first gateway being menarche, the beginning of menstruation, and the last, menopause, the crone or wise woman years). As she is supported by her partner, family, friends, birth attendant, as well as her environment, in *giving* birth to her child, so she taps into the powers of surrender, trust, and selflessness that enable her to mother wisely.

Homeopathy offers the birthing woman a gentle, yet powerful, support to overcome many challenges along the way. It is a natural system of medicine without the side effects often accompanying conventional medical treatment.

The goal of this book is to empower you to use homeopathic medicines safely and effectively during childbirth and the immediate postpartum period even if you are a newcomer to it. It is not meant to replace the midwife or doctor, but to give you a first line of action that can prevent the need for further intervention.

I welcome you to a unique healing approach that will build your self-confidence and understanding of the healing process. Though you are sure to experience many powerful results using the information included, it is only the beginning of what homeopathy has to offer. Homeopathy is a complex science/art that involves a lifetime of study to master. A suggested list of books and resources to continue your study is provided at the end of this book.

For many years, as a midwife, I have been blessed as a witness to, and participant in, the miracle of childbirth. It is clear to me that a woman inherently knows how to give birth when she is given the loving support to believe in herself. I hope this book will assist you to trust and rely on that inner wisdom. Happy birthing!

CHAPTER 1

What Is Homeopathy?

Homeopathy is a form of natural medicine that uses immeasurably small doses of medicines to stimulate the body's own healing ability. It is based on a systematic application of the principles of health and healing. These principles and their application are as true today as they were 200 years ago when homeopathy was developed.

Homeopathy was developed by German physician Samuel Hahnemann (1755 - 1843). Hahnemann became dissatisfied with the conventional medical treatment of his time. So he gave up medical practice and became a medical translator. His curiosity and desire to find the laws of healing led him to experiment with cinchona bark (quinine), which was used then (and is still used today) in conventional medicine to treat malaria. To his surprise, he found that taking very small doses of quinine, until his body reacted to the drug, created in him similar symptoms as those suffering from malaria. Hahnemann continued to perform meticulous drug tests called "provings" to bring out what symptoms different substances cause in a healthy person.

This was the beginning of the medical application of what is known as "The Law of Similars." This law states that a substance can cure a disease if it produces in a healthy person symptoms similar to those of the disease; like is cured by like. It is a law of nature that was earlier recognized by both Hippocrates and Paracelsus. Hahnemann was the first to test the principle systematically and establish it as the foundation of a system of medicine.

Hahnemann continued his testing to discover how small a dose of a drug could be given to stimulate the healing response and yet eliminate the toxic effect. He developed a process known as "potentization," which involves successive dilution alternating with succussion (vigorous shaking) or trituration (grinding). These small doses are called "potencies." Potentization renders medicines nontoxic and without side effects while increasing their potential for cure.

Homeopathy is a truly holistic system of medicine. It recognizes that all parts of the body, as well as the mind and emotions, are interdependent. Therefore, all symptoms of the person are taken into account in order to find the single curative medicine.

Homeopathy aims to restore the individual to a greater overall state of health, vitality, and freedom. Symptoms of disease, according to the homeopathic philosophy of healing, represent the body's best effort to heal itself. Symptoms are seen as positive, adaptive responses to the various stresses experienced by the individual. Therefore, homeopathy does not suppress symptoms; it stimulates the body's overall defenses or vitality to complete the curative process. The result, in most cases, is the elimination of the symptoms of disease along with an improvement in overall health.

Today, homeopathic medicines (remedies) are prepared by homeopathic pharmacies as specified in the

"Homeopathic Pharmacopoeia of the United States," the official manufacturing manual recognized by the FDA. Most remedies are made from plants, but minerals, metals, animal venoms and by-products, as well as chemical drugs are used. Remedies are prepared in the form of small sugar pellets, lactose tablets, or liquid.

Homeopathic remedies are inexpensive and safe to use. The layperson can learn to effectively handle many common nonemergency illnesses for which they would usually seek conventional medical care. It is well suited for those who want to assume greater personal responsibility for their health.

Homeopathy is practiced in nearly every country in the world. It is particularly popular in England, France, India, Mexico, Brazil, Argentina, and the former U.S.S.R. The English Royal Family has been under the care of homeopathic physicians since the 1930's. Two hundred years of worldwide, successful clinical experience continues to prove homeopathy safe and effective in the treatment and prevention of disease.

The history of homeopathy in the United States is a fascinating one. It was extremely popular here in the nineteenth century. The first national medical association of any kind was the American Institute of Homeopathy, founded in 1844. By the turn of the century, one out of four physicians used homeopathy. There were 22 homeopathic medical schools and over 100 homeopathic hospitals. Then came homeopathy's decline in the United States due to a number of factors. These included the acceptance of a more mechanical, as opposed to holistic, view of disease and the body; advances in surgical and pharmaceutical medicine;

strong opposition by the A.M.A. (American Medical Association, founded in 1846) whose Code of Ethics prohibited members from consulting with homeopathic physicians and whose orthodox physicians influenced the passage of legislation detrimental to homeopathic training and practice; as well as infighting among homeopaths regarding doctrine and politics. Today, homeopathy is again experiencing a tremendous resurgence in popularity due to renewed interest in the natural laws of healing, as well as disillusionment with standard medical treatment.

The information presented in this book will, step-by-step, give you access to the safe and effective use of homeopathy and its potential for supporting the birth process.

CHAPTER 2

Remedies to Have in Your Homeopathic Birth Kit

Before the birth, one person should be decided on to be responsible for prescribing remedies during labor. This could be a professional homeopath, the birth attendant, the pregnant woman's partner, or anyone willing to assume and prepare for that role. The birthing woman will be too busy during labor to prescribe for herself. Solicit this person's help in putting the homeopathic birth kit together and choosing the remedies to include. This will give him/her the opportunity to become more familiar with the expectant mother, her individual needs, the homeopathic remedies, and their uses. When possible, it is also a good idea to have a professional homeopath on call to consult with if the need arises.

The remedies listed below are the ones that are most commonly used during birth. However, other remedies may be needed to suit the individual. If the pregnant woman has had other children, thought should be given to her past births and what challenging situations came up. Also think about how she usually responds to pain and stress, mentally, emotionally, and physically. Include in the kit the appropriate remedies from the list suggested below that will cover these situations. You may want to ask a professional homeopath for other remedy suggestions if none of the remedies I have included fits her individual situation or pattern of response.

If the pregnant woman is seeing a professional homeopath and knows what her constitutional remedy is, it should be on hand. A dose of it may be all that she needs.

The remedies in bold type (or bold face) are those one should always include in any basic birthing first-aid kit.

The remedies in plain type are commonly used remedies for birth.

The remedies in italics are not as frequently needed. Read about them and decide if you want to include them in your birth kit.

Aconitum napellus (Aconite) 200c
Antimonium tartaricum 200c
Arnica montana (Arnica) 30c and 200c
Arsenicum album (Arsenicum) 200c
Belladonna 200c
Bellis perennis 30c
Calendula 30c
Calendula tincture, nonalcoholic, or succus
Camphora 200c
Cantharis 200c
Carbo vegetabilis 200c
Caulophyllum 30c and 200c
Chamomilla 200c
China officinalis (China or Cinchona) 200c
Cimicifuga 30c and 200c
Cinnamonum 200c

Coffea cruda (Coffea) 200c
Crotalus horridus 200c
Digitalis 200c
Gelsemium 30c or 200c
Gossypium 30c and 200c
Hamamelis 200c
Hypericum 30c
Ignatia 30c or 200c
Ipecacuanha 200c
Kali carbonicum 30c
Kali phosphoricum 6x
Lachesis 200c
Laurocerasus 200c
Ledum palustre (Ledum) 30c and 200c
Millefolium 200c
Natrum muriaticum 200c
Nux vomica 30c or 200c
*Opium 200c
Phosphorus 200c
Platina 200c
Pulsatilla 200c
Pyrogenium 200c
Rescue Remedy
Sabina 200c
Secale cornutum (Secale) 200c
Sepia 200c
Staphysagria 30c
Trillium 200c
Ustilago maydis (Ustilago) 200c

*No longer available in the U.S. due to the F.D.A. although it is totally safe in homeopathic form.

CHAPTER 3

How to Use
Homeopathic Remedies

Homeopathy is a safe and powerful tool to have as one of many in your bag of tricks. In each chapter, I have tried to give an overall understanding of the topic covered, plus many different approaches that can be helpful. Homeopathic remedies should be used along with the other recommendations. (Note: This book is written for pregnant women, homeopaths, *and* birth attendants. Some chapters, however, such as "Postpartum Hemorrhage," or "Retained Placenta," are meant primarily for the birth attendant or the person prescribing homeopathic remedies for the birthing woman. I suggest that you read all chapters, but concentrate primarily on those parts that apply to your specific role in the birth process.)

Homeopathic remedies are safe for use during pregnancy and birth, if used with common sense. In fact, this is an ideal time for homeopathic care. Nature provides a pregnant woman with tremendous amounts of vital energy in order to grow a healthy baby. Because of this she will respond quickly and clearly when the correctly chosen remedy is taken. Homeopathy can increase her level of health, giving her more vitality, and thus increase the health of her unborn child. Unlike conventional medicines, homeopathic remedies, when used according to the principles of classical homeopathy, are safe and beneficial for the fetus.

It is very difficult to do harm with homeopathy, but some common sense measures should be followed. *Homeopathy does not take the place of appropriate medical care given by a trained birth attendant.* This book assumes that a well trained birth attendant is making sure the necessary medical attention needed prenatally, during birth, as well as postpartum, is received.

There is a possible danger in taking a homeopathic remedy too often over too long period of time, without indications for its use. If taken in this manner, you can cause the very symptoms that you are trying to cure, or bring on other adverse symptoms. This is called "proving" the remedy. This can be avoided by using the following guidelines: A homeopathic remedy will either work, in which case positive results will be seen fairly quickly, or it will not work, and nothing will happen.

Do *not* continue to take a remedy:

- if the symptoms do not continue to improve with each dose,

- if the symptoms are getting worse with each dose, or

- if other troublesome symptoms are appearing.

Stop taking the remedy once the symptoms prescribed for are markedly improved. The remedy has stimulated the body's own healing process, and this should continue on its own. Read more about this under "Repeating the Dose" below. If you are ever in doubt, consult with a professional homeopath.

Some books advise giving a pregnant woman a homeopathic remedy, or combination of remedies, daily for the last month of pregnancy to help her have an easier labor and birth. If she does not have a previous history or current symptoms that would indicate the use of the remedy, this practice could bring on the very symptoms that it is trying to avoid. For this reason, I believe it is preferable not to use homeopathic remedies routinely over a long period of time without specific indications for their use. (See "Repeating the Dose" below.)

Choosing the Remedy:

As already mentioned, during labor, birth, and the immediate postpartum period, the birthing woman will be too busy and otherwise focused to prescribe homeopathic remedies for herself. Prior to that time, she should designate one person who will be responsible for prescribing remedies for her. This could be her partner, birth attendant, professional homeopath, or anyone willing to assume and prepare for that role. It is a good idea, when possible, to have a professional homeopath on call to consult with if the need arises.

Homeopathic prescribing is based on a holistic approach. Even though the individual may have numerous physical as well as psychological symptoms, she has only *one* underlying imbalance or disease. All parts of the body, as well as the mind and emotions, are interdependent. The one underlying imbalance manifests itself, therefore, in these many symptoms. All symptoms of the person are taken into account in order to understand the complete individual picture, the individual "state."

This "totality of symptoms" or individual "state" is used to find the *one* remedy that is most similar. The use of a single remedy at a time is a basic principle of homeopathy because of this holistic view.

The person prescribing homeopathic remedies needs to answer the following questions: How is she (the birthing woman) responding to her labor, birth, and her environment? What is she feeling? What is her psychological state? What is her mental state like? Is she afraid? If so, of what? What physical symptoms need to be alleviated? What other symptoms accompany the main complaint? What makes her, in general, and her physical symptoms, specifically, better or worse? What is her general state like: sleep, thirst, appetite, body temperature, perspiration, vitality? What sets her apart from other laboring women? What is her individual experience?

You want to match her individual state to the *single* remedy that is most similar. Use those symptoms that are the most intense or unique about the woman you are prescribing for. What makes her stand out as an individual? Often this will indicate the overall mental-emotional response she is experiencing and/or the strong physical symptom you are prescribing for. Do not emphasize symptoms that are common for pregnant and birthing women, such as feeling vulnerable, low sexual desire, feeling hot, more thirsty than usual, and desiring open air, unless these symptoms are particularly intense. Only those symptoms that are unique, unusual, and more intense than usual for that individual will lead you to the correct remedy, because

11

these are the symptoms that show you the individuality of this woman's vitality.

Use the general symptoms (sleep, thirst, appetite, body temperature, perspiration, general vitality, as well as the symptoms of the mental-emotional state) to confirm a remedy or to decide between two different remedies. General symptoms are extremely valuable because they represent the reaction of the whole person, not just a specific part. As such, they represent the deeper level of response in attempting to reestablish health. General symptoms are expressed with such statements as, "*I* feel tired" or "*I* love pickles," rather than "*My* legs hurt," as this refers to a specific part.

General symptoms are subdivided into mental general symptoms and physical general symptoms. Mental general symptoms consist of the symptoms of the mental-emotional state, i.e., irritable, angry, sensitive, weepy, etc. An important general symptom is conveyed by a physical symptom if it represents a reaction *of the whole body*. For example, the lack of uterine tone of *Sepia* can be seen as general sluggishness in the lack of tone of the woman's stomach muscles, constipation, urinary incontinence, possible uterine prolapse, as well as her lack of energy and mood of indifference. Vigorous exercise makes her generally better because it temporarily brings her out of this sluggish state. This sluggishness is a general symptom that expresses itself through numerous physical and mental symptoms.

A homeopathic prescription can also be based on a strong and unusual general symptom(s) or unique physical symptom(s), when the mental-emotional symptoms are mild or even absent. If that particular remedy strongly addresses the symptom you are prescribing for, it is likely to be an effective remedy. For example, *Pulsatilla* has a strong general symptom of changeability. It can be prescribed for the woman whose contractions come and go but who's labor never gets established, based on this changeability. A confirmation of some of the mental-emotional or other general symptoms would be nice, but is not necessary for this prescription to be an effective one.

In the remedy descriptions, I am trying to paint a vivid picture in your mind of what the woman needing that specific remedy would look like, feel like, and sound like. For this reason, as well as to avoid using redundant and lengthy language, I use the name of the remedy to represent the woman needing that remedy. Obviously, a remedy cannot feel or experience. So, for example, when I say, "*Caulophyllum* can look similar to *Pulsatilla*. Both are emotionally soft, sweet, and weepy," I am referring to the woman who will benefit from the use of *Caulophyllum* or *Pulsatilla*. Please do not become confused by this personalization of the remedies.

You will also notice that I refer to specific "types" when describing remedy pictures, i.e., "the *Arsenicum* type," or "the *Pulsatilla* type." While classical homeopathic prescribing is based on the symptoms and state of the individual, it has been noticed that certain types of people (often referred to as "constitutional types") react strongly to certain remedies. Therefore, homeopaths may say, for example, that "the characteristic *Phosphorus* (type) woman is tall, thin, and delicate, with long fingers." This line of thinking has its limitations since, in reality, each person must be considered as an individual. However, for the sake of convenience, you will find similar descriptions included in this book.

Each remedy description represents the "disease" state that can be cured by that same remedy. This is because according to the science of homeopathy, a substance that can produce disease symptoms in a healthy person will, when prepared and used according to homeopathic principles, cure those same symptoms. Therefore, when I write that "*Caulophyllum* has sharp, stitching, cramping pains," or "*Aconite* has sudden, intense attacks of fear with flushed face, heart palpitations, and bounding pulse," you will want to consider that remedy if the woman you are prescribing for has the same symptoms.

I suggest going to the appropriate chapter and reading through it, getting an overall sense of each remedy picture. The individual you are prescribing for will seldom have every symptom in the remedy descriptions. Nor will her mental-emotional state always be as extreme as the one described. Think of the mental-emotional state as a progression from mild to severe. Your individual should fit somewhere along that line, while matching the overall state of the remedy well.

At the end of some of the remedy descriptions, I have included information to help you differentiate between that remedy and others with similar symptoms.

The remedies are listed alphabetically into one or two sections: "First Remedies to Consider," and "Other Remedies to Consider."

There are also repertories in the back of the chapters that have more than five remedies in them. Use them to help you think of the remedies to consider for a particular symptom. (Note: The repertories were compiled mainly from *The Complete Repertory* by Van Zandvoort from *MacRepertory*, the *Synthetic Bedside*

Repertory for Gestation, Childbirth, and Childbed by Jan Jansen, and *The Accoucheur's Emergency Manual* by W.A. Yingling. I have made some additions and upgraded some of the remedies in order to distinguish them for prescribing purposes.) You will also find here the unique characteristic symptoms and matching remedy to help you base a prescription on. For example, a number of remedies are listed under "profuse hemorrhage," but only *Belladonna* has "coagulates quickly, sudden, profuse, and hot" bleeding with the hemorrhage. This is a characteristic symptom for someone needing *Belladonna*.

Do not rule out a particular remedy because it is not listed in the repertory for every symptom of the woman you are prescribing for. Choose those symptoms that are the most immediate, intense, and unique on which to base the prescription. A repertory is only a guide, useful to give suggestions of remedies to consider. Always read the complete remedy descriptions to find the best matching remedy before making your decision.

In the remedy descriptions, the mental-emotional picture is usually first, followed by the physical general symptoms and characteristic (unique) physical symptoms. In some instances where a remedy is prescribed based upon its usefulness for a particular physical symptom, such as *Arnica* for soreness and bruising, or *Caulophyllum* for weak or uncoordinated contractions, only the physical symptoms may be included or emphasized.

When the correct remedy is chosen the curative response is fast and can often seem "miraculous." On the other hand, it can be very frustrating to try a number of remedies without the desired result. Be patient with yourself. This is part of the process of learning homeopathy. With time and experience, the remedies will become like old friends, and you will easily recognize the overall state and specific symptoms that call for their use.

Choosing the Potency:

Homeopathic remedies come in different potencies. I consider 6x, 12x, 30x, 6c, or 12c to be low potencies, 30c to be a medium potency, and 200c or 1M to be a high potency. A 30c is an excellent basic potency to have for most self-care situations, however, for emergencies such as neonatal asphyxia (breathing difficulty in the newborn) or hemorrhage, you will want to have 200c or higher potency on hand. A 200c is also a good potency for the intense phases of birth. Many midwives carry mainly this potency in their homeopathic birth kits.

In general, you want to match the intensity and severity of the situation with the potency. A mild situation will do well with a lower potency and can be repeated as needed. Using a high potency will be better for a more intense or severe situation. The vitality required for a severe situation uses up the remedy more quickly. A high potency will be effective for a longer period of time and does not need to be repeated often. With a lower potency you will have to repeat the dose more often.

Don't get too hung up on the potency. The golden rule for choosing a potency is, *the correct potency to use is the one you have on hand.* Choosing the correct remedy is more important than choosing the correct potency.

How to Take the Remedy:

Homeopathic remedies come in the form of different sized pellets or tablets. They can be taken dry under the tongue or dissolved in water and taken a spoonful at a time, as needed.

The amount or size of the dose in homeopathy is not as important as it is with conventional pharmaceuticals. A baby can swallow a whole vial of a homeopathic medicine and it is the same as taking one dose of the remedy. There is no danger.

I usually recommend as one dose:

- 2 medium sized pellets (size of peppercorns) OR

- 5 very small pellets (size of mustard seeds) OR

- 1 or 2 tablets OR

- Add one pellet or tablet to about 4 ounces of water, stir vigorously 15 – 20 times, and take one teaspoon. The remedy does not need to be dissolved before you take a dose. Stir vigorously again before each dose. Cover the cup with a clean piece of paper between doses.

Carefully tip the pellets or tablets into the lid of the bottle. If more than the desired number falls out, tip the others back into the bottle without touching them. Then tip the pellets or tablets from the lid into the mouth, preferably under the tongue, and let them dissolve there. Do not touch the lid with the mouth or tongue. Replace the lid on the bottle.

It is important not to contaminate the bottle of

remedy with surface bacteria or other substances. Never put back pellets or tablets that have fallen out onto the floor or anywhere else, or that have been touched by you or anyone else. Throw these away.

For a newborn, the dose is the same as for an adult. To prevent possible gagging or spitting out of the remedy, you can crush a dose between 2 clean spoons and place the resulting powder into her mouth. The water method mentioned above can also be used. This method is especially convenient if the dose needs to be frequently repeated. (Note: My apologies for choosing to use the female pronouns "she" and "her" to represent all newborns. The English language does not offer a gracious or appropriate alternative. "He" has been overly used. "It" is offensive to me.)

Avoid putting anything into the mouth 10 minutes before and 10 minutes after taking the remedy. Plain water is O.K. to drink if absolutely necessary. This can be difficult during labor when the birthing woman needs to stay hydrated while perhaps needing a remedy often. Do the best that you can within the circumstances. This rule does not apply to breast-feeding newborns.

Do not use the following while under homeopathic care because they can totally interfere with the action of homeopathic remedies:

- coffee (even decaffeinated, since it's the coffee bean, not the caffeine, you want to avoid);

- camphor or camphorated products such as Vick's Vaporub, Noxema, Ben Gay, Tiger Balm, Carmex, some types of Blistex, etc.;

- eucalyptus, tea tree oil, strong incense, perfumes or moth balls;

- electric blankets; unplug the electric blanket after heating the bed;

- recreational drugs such as marijuana.

Repeating the Dose:

As mentioned in the opening chapter, a homeopathic remedy acts to stimulate the body's own healing response. Therefore, it is not necessary to continue giving the remedy once the healing response has been catalyzed. In homeopathy, *more is not better.* The ideal is to give a remedy only as much as is needed to stimulate the healing response, then repeat it only when and if the original symptoms you based your prescription on are beginning to return. There are, however, basic guidelines that are helpful to remember:

For *mild* situations (i.e., postpartum healing, such as soreness, bruising, perineal tears):

- Use a 30c potency 3 – 4 times a day. If the prescription is correct, marked improvement should be noticed within 24 hours.

For *moderate* situations, when you need to know fairly quickly if the remedy is correct (i.e., most labor situations such as dysfunctional labor, back labor, and postpartum pain):

- Use a 30c potency every 15 minutes for an hour, every hour for 3 hours, then 3 times a day for several days, or as needed. A curative response should be noticed within the first hour (first 4 doses) with the correct remedy.

- For excruciating pain, a 30c can be given every few minutes, for a few doses, then as needed for the pain. You should notice less pain after the first few doses, and after each subsequent dose. Each dose should be effective for a longer period of time.

- 200c is a good potency for the intense phases of labor and birth. Many midwives carry mainly this potency in their homeopathic birth kits. Use it when you are fairly sure of your prescription, or if the 30c potency has been working well and then stops being effective. A healing response should be seen soon after a single dose of a 200c. It may need to be repeated once or twice again if the symptoms return.

In *emergency* situations, such as neonatal asphyxia or postpartum hemorrhage:

- Use a 200c potency. The response will be almost immediate with the right remedy. Repeat the remedy up to every 10 seconds and change it if there is no response after 2 doses. Stop giving the remedy when the symptoms improve, or if there is no improvement after 2 doses. Repeat the remedy only if the original symptoms return.

- If 30c is what is on hand for an emergency situation, repeat it as with the 200c potency.

Improvement should be seen rapidly with the correct remedy.

Taking Care of Homeopathic Remedies:

Homeopathic remedies will keep their strength indefinitely if they are properly stored.

- Keep them in a cool, dry, and dark place.

- Keep them away from strong smelling odors, especially camphor, tea tree oil, perfumes, and mothballs. For this reason, it is not a good idea to keep them in a medicine cabinet.

- Keep the remedy vials out of direct sunlight or very high heat (120° or higher), which can deactivate the remedies.

- Screw the lids on tightly immediately after dispensing the remedy to avoid contamination.

- Again, if any of the remedy falls on the floor or anywhere else, or is touched by yourself or someone else, throw it away. Do not put it back in the remedy vial.

CHAPTER *4*

Inducing Labor

Labor naturally begins due to an intricate interplay between mother and baby. Though the details of this interplay are not clearly understood, it is evident that what best maintains the physical and emotional health of both mother and child is the support of the natural process.

Today, unfortunately, many labors are induced unnecessarily. Though there are times when the artificial induction of labor is warranted, these are rare. Make sure that if induction of labor is considered, it is only when it is truly indicated for maintaining the health of mother and baby.

The main reason that labor is unnecessarily induced is because the due date is incorrect. The due date should be calculated from the first day of the last menstrual cycle. That cycle should have been normal, lasting as many days as usual, and with as much flow as usual, not just a spotting episode.

The last menstrual period is the most accurate gauge for dating; however, if the date of the last period is uncertain, it is probably a good idea to have an ultrasound in order to avoid undue anxiety about a possible postdates situation. I do not recommend ultrasounds during the first trimester, if possible, because this is the time when the baby is forming all her vital systems. Though ultrasound is generally considered to be safe, there are still unknowns as to its overall effect. Therefore, waiting until the second trimester (13 weeks) is a prudent choice.

Keep in mind that an ultrasound is more accurate for dating the earlier it is done (although I do not recommend one before 13 weeks, as explained above). It is most accurate (plus or minus one week) if done before 22 weeks gestation, less accurate (plus or minus 2 weeks) if done at 22 – 28 weeks gestation, and highly inaccurate if done after 28 weeks gestation. This is because in the third trimester, the fetus begins to grow in her own unique pattern. So an ultrasound done in the last trimester of pregnancy is basically useless for dating.

At 41 weeks, there is concern regarding the healthy functioning of the placenta, the organ responsible for physically nourishing the baby in utero. The life of the placenta is approximately 42 weeks, after which it begins to break down, no longer nourishing the baby properly. There are simple tests, such as the Non-Stress Test (NST) or Biophysical Profile, that can be done beginning at 41 weeks, letting you know if the placenta is doing its job. They should be repeated weekly until labor begins. Talk to your care provider about where to have these test performed.

Pitocin is the synthetic hormone used to induce labor. Even with great sensitivity by the practitioner monitoring the induction, the contractions produced with pitocin are more painful than those of natural labor, making the labor more difficult to deal with for both mother and baby. This often leads to a whole chain of problems and interventions. Therefore, it is best whenever possible to begin labor naturally.

The first and most important step I recommend when you want to get labor started is to encourage the pregnant woman and her partner (if she has one) to sit down and have a heart-to-heart talk in a quiet, safe environment in order to clear any emotional obstacles that may be in the way. (Note: Though I am addressing the pregnant woman and her partner in doing this process, it can also effectively be done with the labor support person, a close friend, or as a gestalt dialogue with herself.) It is important that neither feel accused or judged while doing this clearing. The couple should present helpful suggestions to each other gently instead of as criticisms. There must be complete honesty and safety for this process to be effective. Any emotions that come up must be allowed to fully express and clear themselves. Tears are cleansing and these feelings will not hurt the baby. They are being release. Encourage each partner to go deeply and explore every possible thought or fear, however silly or embarrassing. As much time as needed to feel complete must be taken, maybe continuing tomorrow, if need be.

The following is a list of suggested areas to explore:

- Are we ready for this baby to join our lives?

- Does anything need to happen first?

- Is our home ready?

- Is there anything to clear up in ourselves, our relationship, or with someone else?

- If there are any other siblings, are they ready

for the arrival of their new brother or sister?

- How do we feel about the upcoming birth?

- Are there any fears that need to be dealt with?

- Are we ready to let go of the pregnancy (perhaps it's the last planned pregnancy)?

- Are we reluctant to give up the special attention we are enjoying during pregnancy?

- Are we afraid of the responsibilities of parenting?

- How much trust do we feel for my body and its ability to safely birth our baby? (Creative visualizations of the upcoming birth might be useful here. There are some excellent audio and videotapes available for this purpose. Ask a midwife or childbirth educator for recommendations.)

- Are there any feelings from past experiences that need to be dealt with and cleared up first (a past abortion, miscarriage, adoption, birth experience)?

- Was our own birth difficult and do we need to clear these feelings? (Birth memories are often relived at an unconscious level during birthing. I suggest, if possible, that the couple talk to their mothers about their own births to find out what happened. Rebirthing is a very useful technique for clearing out these memories and for opening to the positive energy of birth.)

- Do we trust our birth attendant and feel safe

25

with the people who will be there?

- "Check in" with the unborn child and find out if there is anything she needs to express or have done before she is ready to be born.

This is just a sample of areas that may need to be explored. Clearing should continue until all emotionally charged areas have been fully looked into.

Be sure to have her access her wise part (we all have one) for any further thoughts, feelings, and suggestions. Encourage her to find her center, tap into her inner strength and clarity, and trust the inner guidance that comes through. Thoughts and emotions are extremely powerful, and just airing them helps them to clear. Since body and mind work together, this process is often all that is needed to allow labor to begin.

If the pregnant woman is seeing a professional homeopath for chronic care, consult with them to see if another or stronger dose of the constitutional remedy is needed, or if another specific remedy is indicated.

Now is the time for her to nurture and refresh herself. This may mean quiet time to think, feel, and reflect, getting regular massages, bodywork, chiropractic adjustments, doing yoga, doing deep breathing and relaxation exercises, going out to dinner, spending more time with her partner and/or children, getting lots of sleep, etc.

Other methods that help bring on labor are going for long, brisk walks, going for long rides on a bumpy road, stimulating the breasts, particularly the nipples (triggers the release of oxytocin, the hormone which causes contractions), and lovemaking (semen has prostaglandins which soften and prepare the cervix).

If the midwife finds that the cervical opening is tight and rigid, or if there is scar tissue there from recent infections or surgery, try massaging some evening primrose oil (available at health food stores) on the cervix once or twice a day. A cervix that is not ready for labor will feel thick, firm, and about an inch long. A "ripe" cervix feels softer, mushier, with a less distinguishable neck of only half an inch or so. Evening primrose oil will soften the tissue, break up adhesions, and prepare the cervix to dilate. She can also take 3 – 6 capsules a day orally. This can also be done in early labor, in case it is prolonged.

Remember that patience, letting go, and trusting is definitely the name of the game in the last days or weeks of pregnancy. After she has done all that she can, just plain forgetting about it may be what will help her relax the most. If she is sure of her dates, her cervix is ripe, the baby appears to be term (by estimated size and recent growth pattern), labor still hasn't started, and the midwife is getting concerned, it's time to move on and get more aggressive.

First Remedies to Consider:

This is the protocol I generally use to help bring on labor:

> *Caulophyllum* 30c or 200c alternating with *Cimicifuga* 30c or 200c every 2 hours for 6 total doses in 24 hours. No remedy the next day. Repeat the same protocol on day 3 if needed.

This protocol is very powerful, but will only work if the pregnant woman's body and the baby are ready for birth. Otherwise, it will help tone her uterus and prepare her for the upcoming birth. No harm done!

Other Remedies to Consider:

Gelsemium: Excellent remedy when there is fear of birth. It is used commonly to initiate labor. The woman who will benefit from *Gelsemium* fears challenging tasks. She fears that she will not be able to persist and accomplish the birth. She tends to be emotionally timid, perhaps trembling with nervous or emotional excitement in anticipation of all that is to come. She feels weak, tired, and fearful in anticipation of labor and birth.

Read more about *Gelsemium* in the chapter "Prolonged, Difficult, or Dysfunctional Labor."

Pulsatilla: A useful remedy when contractions come and go, but labor never gets established. Changeability is a strong general symptom of *Pulsatilla*, and can be the basis for your choice of this remedy. Give a dose of *Pulsatilla* 200c every two hours for up to three doses. The contractions will either stop (if her body and the baby are not ready for birth), or labor will begin in earnest. Some midwives and homeopaths alternate *Pulsatilla* and *Caulophyllum* (as described above for *Caulophyllum* and *Cimicifuga*) to induce labor.

Pulsatilla is particularly indicated for the woman who has a strong need for affection, attention, approval, and reassurance from others. Her emotions are on the surface. She is easily moved to tears and feels much better from crying. She tends to be soft, sweet, affectionate, and sympathetic. She wants plenty of fresh air and will have the windows wide open.

Read more about *Pulsatilla* in the chapter "Prolonged, Difficult, or Dysfunctional Labor."

Homeopathy and acupuncture are both energetic medicines. Since they affect the same deep levels, one may interfere with the action of the other. Therefore, it is generally not recommended to receive acupuncture treatment while you are under homeopathic care. With this in mind, however, I mention acupuncture here as an option to be considered if the remedies and methods recommended in this chapter have not been effective and the pregnant woman is not under constitutional homeopathic care. This warning does not generally apply to acupressure and moxibustion. (Note: Acupressure involves applying external pressure at the acupuncture points. Moxibustion uses the heat of burning "moxa," the compressed dried leaves of Chinese mugwort, applied at the acupuncture points. Both methods are used to stimulate acupuncture points without the insertion of needles.)

The following acupressure technique can be used in conjunction with the other methods suggested in this chapter. Chinese acupuncture point Spleen 6 (Sp6) is known as the "labor point" because it helps to bring on labor and strengthen contractions. It is located 3 fingerwidths above the anklebone on the inside of the leg and a little forward in the hollow between the lower leg bones. Locate that general spot and feel around until you find the most tender spot. That's it! Apply firm pressure 10 minutes at a time. Seeing a professional acupressurist or acupuncturist can also be helpful. They will use moxa or acupuncture needles to more strongly stimulate Spleen 6 and other points.

The use of castor oil is the last method I consider to induce labor. The sensations are unpleasant because it causes urgent bowel movements that continue even after the bowels are empty. However, castor oil induction is usually effective, safer, and more pleasant than pitocin induction, therefore it is well worth it. Keep it in mind when all other methods have not started labor, pitocin induction seems inevitable, and everything else appears normal. Be sure the baby's head is either engaged or very low in the pelvis because there is a small risk of rupture of the membranes which could cause the cord to prolapse if the baby's head is high. Have the midwife check the fetal heart tones when labor begins to make sure the baby is handling the contractions well.

After the pregnant woman is well rested, have her take 2 ounces of castor oil in 2 or more ounces of orange juice. Wait an hour and repeat the same dose. Taking a hot shower or bath will help her to relax. Labor may begin right away or can take up to 6 hours to get going. (Note: Though I am normally comfortable with a laboring woman bathing in her own tub, I do not recommend a bath if the membranes are ruptured and she is not in active labor or she is using castor oil, because of the increased possibility of infection.)

In the highly unlikely event that the woman is still faced with pitocin induction and if time permits, ask the doctor to first use prostaglandin gel (locally applied to the cervix). This will often begin labor without the pitocin, and, worse case, will greatly increase the effectiveness of the pitocin induction by ripening the cervix.

CHAPTER 5

Changing the Baby's Presentation Prior to Labor

The most favorable presentation for a baby to be born in is head first (vertex), with the back side lying towards the front of the mother. Other presentations and positions can lengthen labor, be more difficult, and hold more risks of complications. Breech presentations (baby born bottom first) are often routinely delivered via cesarean section, though vaginal birth is a definite option with a birth attendant who is experienced in such deliveries.

Breeches can, on their own, rotate to vertex right up to the time that labor starts. However, as the baby grows, there is less and less room for them to maneuver in. It is a good idea to encourage a breech to turn beginning at about 32 weeks gestation.

The first method to use is the tilt position. Have the pregnant woman lie on her back on the floor, with knees flexed, feet on the floor, and hips about twelve inches off the floor (by placing three or so good-sized pillows under her bottom). This is done for 10 – 20 minutes twice a day. She should be as relaxed as possible, do deep relaxation breathing, and visualize the baby turning. She can also very gently massage the baby, if she knows in what direction she needs to go to turn. When she feels the baby turning head down, she should get up and go for a long walk. This will help the head to settle deeply in her pelvis.

First Remedy to Consider:

Homeopathy can help a baby to turn. The following protocol works well for many women. Try it when she is 35 to 36 weeks gestation, preferably before the baby's presenting part is engaged:

> *Pulsatilla* 30c, one dose every two hours for up to 6 doses in 24 hours, or *Pulsatilla* 200c once. Nothing the next day and repeat the same dosage on the third day, if necessary. Discontinue sooner when the baby turns.

If the above protocol is not successful, she may need to see a professional homeopath to prescribe a specific remedy for her and her baby.

Another Remedy to Consider:

Natrum muriaticum: Useful for turning a baby when you suspect the position is due to too little amniotic fluid, particularly if the woman matches the overall picture of this remedy.

Read more about *Natrum muriaticum* in the chapter "Prolonged, Difficult, or Dysfunctional Labor."

There is a method in Chinese medicine that is also very effective for changing a baby's position. This involves stimulation of the acupuncture point Urinary Bladder 67 (B67). B67 is located at the outside corner of the tip of the baby toe, next to the toenail. Stimulate this point with firm pressure for 10 to 15 minutes. Seeing a professional acupressurist or acupuncturist can also be helpful, as they can stimulate B67 more strongly with moxa or acupuncture needles. (Note: Read my warning about the use of acupuncture while under homeopathic care in the chapter, "Inducing Labor.")

There is the rare baby who needs to remain in her present position for some unknown reason. These babies tend to do fine delivering in that position. Discuss the safety and possibility of delivering the baby breech with a midwife experienced in such deliveries.

A final option is to have the midwife or physician perform an external version, where an attempt is made to manually turn the baby. It is usually done in the hospital with the aid of a muscle relaxant and ultrasound. *Be sure the midwife or physician is skilled at this technique.* It is a somewhat aggressive, but usually safe, approach that should not be tried except as a last resort. Even with a successful version, some babies turn right back around. Again, these babies need to remain in their position for some unknown reason, and they tend to do fine delivering in that position.

CHAPTER 6

False Labor (Preparatory Labor)

I prefer to call this preparatory labor because there is nothing false about it. Each contraction is preparing the uterus for the more intense labor that is coming. Each contraction completed now is one less contraction that needs to occur later on. Each does its job.

Since these contractions are relatively mild, it is an excellent time to learn to relax with each one, letting them do their job of opening up the cervix. This surrendering to the process of labor is easier if it is begun now.

When a contraction begins, have the woman take a deep cleansing breath, blowing out all tension. She should continue to gently and deeply breathe in relaxation through her nose and breathe out tension through her mouth. As she does this, she can mentally run through her body checking to be sure that her jaw is relaxed and very loose, her lips are loose, her shoulders are low and relaxed, her lower back is relaxed, and her bottom and thighs are loose. As the contraction ends, she can take another deep cleansing breath. (This is the basic breathing pattern most women find will successfully carry them through most of their labor.) When she has gotten the knack of this breathing and relaxation pattern, she can just forget about it. Let it be automatic, only checking in to make adjustments if any tension is noticed.

Make sure she is well nourished, well hydrated, and well rested. This will pay off later on when she needs to draw upon her reserves.

Read the chapter "Inducing Labor" about clearing feelings and the other methods that apply to help strengthen labor.

CHAPTER 7

Prolonged, Difficult, or Dysfunctional Labor

The length of labor is very unique and individual. It is impossible to fit every labor into a set pattern, though that is what is attempted in most hospitals. The important factors to monitor are that the baby is handling the contractions well, the mother is well hydrated, not overly exhausted, in a good frame of mind, dealing with the contractions effectively, and is making some progress.

There are ebbs and flows in all natural processes. This is also true for labor. Some pauses are the body's wise way of letting a woman rest up before going on with the hard work she is doing. This is particularly true at about 3 – 4 centimeters dilation, 7 centimeters dilation (prior to transition), and when she is completely dilated (10 centimeters) and preparing to push her baby out.

When things slow down, it is important to check in and clear any negative or ambivalent thoughts or feelings there might be. Even if she has done a good job of clearing her fears already, new ones may crop up for the laboring woman along the way. Keep checking in and clearing as need be. Just verbalizing how she feels can be incredibly powerful.

Checks need to be made outside too. Is anything going on that is upsetting her? Are people there who don't need to be? I can't say enough about how important it is for her to feel safe, secure, and nurtured by the environment and the people there. Don't be overly concerned about hurting someone's feelings if you need to ask them to leave. What is important is the well-being of the birthing woman and her baby *right now*, and they should understand this. It is a good idea to have one person she trusts assigned the job of keeping the environment safe for her, so she doesn't have to think about this while in labor.

Be sure she is drinking at least half a cup of juice (diluted 1/2 water, 1/2 juice) or tea sweetened with honey every hour to keep herself hydrated and her energy up. Suggest changes in her position if things aren't progressing. During contractions, she can try squatting, or the hands and knees position. Walking, dancing, going outside for a refreshing walk with her partner, taking a relaxing bath or shower, etc., can also make a difference. It may even be appropriate for her to take a nap, if she can, or just completely relax and drift off between contractions to refresh herself. Sometimes the body wisely slows things down or even completely stops labor (very common at full dilation before the urge to push begins), giving the woman a chance to rest and gather her energy. Keep her energy fresh and upbeat. Make changes well before exhaustion sets in. An exhausted uterus does not work well and is at risk of hemorrhaging after birth.

Read the chapter "Back Labor and Posterior Position of the Baby" for help with an arrested labor due to posterior position of the baby.

First Remedies to Consider:

(Note: Remember that in order to paint a vivid picture in your mind of the woman who would benefit from a particular remedy, as well as to avoid redundant language, I have written about the remedies as if they have human qualities. Refer back to the section, "Choosing the Remedy," in the chapter, "How To Use Homeopathic Remedies," for a further explanation.)

Caulophyllum (Blue cohosh): A powerful labor enhancer and regulator. Will often bring on active labor. Useful to coordinate and strengthen contractions.

The woman who will benefit from *Caulophyllum* tends to be weak and exhausted and so are her contractions. Her contractions are painful, spasmodic, uncoordinated, short in duration, and change locations. Strong contractions seem to have no effect because they are centered in the lower segment of the uterus, instead of the fundus. The contractions come and go, and move from one place to another. The pains may radiate to the bladder, groin or lower extremities, and may feel like pricking of needles in the cervix. Labor does not progress. The vaginal examination shows that the cervical os is very rigid and not stretchy.

There is marked weakness, muscular exhaustion, and trembling (see *Gelsemium*). There is chilliness with shivering, even when she is covered up. She is exhausted out of proportion to the work she has done in labor. The *Caulophyllum* woman tends to be soft, sweet, tearful and delicate (see *Pulsatilla*). She does not want to talk though she wants others around her. There may be nervousness and moody irritability (not anger) with the exhaustion. She is just exhausted and unable to muster the strength necessary for the effort of labor.

Caulophyllum is useful for stalled labors with weak contractions when there are no other symptoms to confirm the use of another remedy. Think of it in premature labor when the waters have broken and the contractions are absent or weak. Think of it also when labor has been going well with strong contractions, then because labor is prolonged, she becomes exhausted and weak, and the contractions become weak and irregular.

Caulophyllum can look similar to *Pulsatilla*. Both are emotionally soft, sweet, and weepy. Both have changeable moods and want people around them. Both desire fresh open air, wanting the windows open. *Caulophyllum*, however, is not as emotionally expressive as *Pulsatilla*, nor as needy for attention and affection. In general, the *Caulophyllum* woman tends to be more chilly, sensitive to cold, and thirsty.

Caulophyllum, in general, have a milder disposition than *Cimicifuga*. The *Caulophyllum* woman is not as energetic or hysterical with the pains. She is softer and not as talkative. Her trembling is more from weakness whereas *Cimicifuga's* is more from nervousness. Some midwives alternate *Caulophyllum* with *Cimicifuga* 12c or 30c to augment labor, if there is not a clear picture for one or the other. Read about *Cimicifuga* below.

The trembling weakness is similar to *Gelsemium*. *Gelsemium*, however, is more drowsy and there is no thirst. Think of *Gelsemium* when *Caulophyllum* seems indicated with the trembling weakness, but fails to work.

Cimicifuga (*Black cohosh*): Helps produce coordinated contractions while allaying fear and anxiety. Helps the

Cimicifuga woman to trust the birth process and to open up, both emotionally and physically (see *Natrum muriaticum*).

The woman needing *Cimicifuga* feels trapped with no way out. She is afraid of the birth and that something terrible is going to happen. She may fear death (see *Aconite*), going crazy, or being poisoned. She feels overly sensitive and unable to endure labor. Common statements are "I can't do it" or, "I can't take it anymore." She is sad, depressed, fearful, pessimistic, and has gloomy states where she sits silently and sighs, as if a black cloud has settled over her. Alternately, there is loquaciousness with a tendency to jump from one subject to another. She is restless, excitable, hysterical, and continuously talking about her complaints, worries and fears. This is accompanied by sighing. Everything seems wrong in her life and she is dissatisfied with whatever you do for her. There is shivering and nervous trembling.

A terrifying or unbearably painful memory of a past pregnancy, birth, miscarriage, or abortion that returns to haunt her may be the cause of the deep gloominess and disabling fear (see *Ignatia*). This could also be from a past history of sexual abuse. The deep fear may not be volunteered or easily elicited, as she may be guarding even herself from it. She, therefore, is fragmented and her gestures, speech, and actions may appear disjointed. Physical symptoms alternate back and forth with one another or with mental or emotional states in an abrupt, jumbled, and random fashion. This can be frightening to her and to those observing, as she appears to be coming "unglued."

Like *Caulophyllum*, *Cimicifuga* has sharp, stitching, cramping pains that are changeable, come and go, and sometimes radiate. The *Cimicifuga* woman has pains which are felt in the lower uterine segment and cervix, which fails to dilate. The pains shoot from side to side or into hips and thighs. They double her up. She is intolerant of the pain, cries out, and says she can't do it. Both cervical regions (cervical os and the upper cervicals or neck) are rigid and stiff. The cervical os dilates, then suddenly constricts spasmodically. Every little distraction will stop the contractions.

She is oversensitive to noise, chilly, has chills with the contractions, and may restlessly toss about. The physical symptoms alternate with mental and emotional symptoms.

Cimicifuga is more hysterical and disjointed than *Caulophyllum*, as are the *Cimicifuga* woman's symptoms. She is more nervous, has more fears, and is more intolerant to pain. The pains tend to be more violent. She is agitated and more energetic with the pains, perhaps even screaming. There is sighing. The cervical os is not as rigid. There can be cramping all over her body (hips, back, and neck).

Cimicifuga can look like *Ignatia* because of the hysterical tendency, the sighing, the crying, the negativity, and the ailments arising from grief. *Ignatia*, however, tends to be more reserved and does not show her deeper feelings as easily. The *Cimicifuga* woman is more excitable and open, talking loquaciously about her complaints. Her grief can lead to frightful premonitions of insanity, from a fragmented and dissociated state.

Read more about *Ignatia* in this chapter and also in the chapter "Healing From a Difficult Delivery or Cesarean Section."

I have seen *Cimicifuga* work wonders in stalled

41

labors where the feelings of gloom and discourage-
ment were mild and not evident to me at the time. The
following personal account illustrates one such experience. Stephanie had planned to birth her baby at
home. She seemed happy and excited about the pros-
pect of labor and birth, though her previous birth had
been long and arduous. After 2 days, Stephanie's contractions continued to be mild and about 10 minutes
apart. She was getting fatigued and wanted labor to
progress. I gave her *Caulophyllum*, which helped within
minutes to bring on stronger contractions about every
5 minutes. However, her labor pattern again stayed
the same for a number of hours and *Caulophyllum* had
no further affect. One dose of *Cimicifuga* 200c did the
trick. Within 15 minutes her contractions went from 5
minutes apart to 3 minutes apart, and she progressed
rapidly from there on. After the birth, Stephanie and I
realized that her fears had definitely been there, though
unexpressed, and stemmed from her past difficult birth
experience. I have also used *Cimicifuga* successfully
when a long labor slows down after little progress, and
the thought of transporting to the hospital from a home
environment had everyone discouraged.

Caulophyllum is my first thought for weak, irregular contractions, without other symptoms, then *Cimicifuga*. Some midwives alternate *Caulophyllum* with
Cimicifuga 12c or 30c to augment labor, if there is not a
clear picture for one or the other.

Other Remedies to Consider:

Aconite: Extreme fear of death during labor, either
from imagined or real circumstances, leads us to this
remedy.

The woman needing *Aconite* has sudden, intense attacks of fear with flushed face, heart palpitations, and bounding pulse. She says, "I'm going to die," and predicts the time of death. She fears that something is going to happen to the baby (see *Arsenicum*). There is great fear and restlessness with each pain. The pains are violent and frightful. Labor fails to progress due to fear. The cervical os contracts spasmodically. She is intolerant of, and extremely sensitive to, a vaginal exam.

This state can be brought on from fright or after exposure to cold wind. She is very thirsty for cold drinks, is aggravated in a warm room, and feels better from open air.

Though *Aconite* may be needed at any time during labor and birth, it is of particular use during transition (the last part of first stage of labor when a woman goes from 8 centimeters dilation to complete dilation). During transition, labor is normally very fast and intense with one contraction coming on top of another. This can cause the *Aconite* woman to be extremely anxious and fearful, feeling that things are out of control and that something horrible is about to happen. *Aconite* will help to calm her sense of panic so she can regain her center.

Aconite is also wonderful for fathers or others at the labor and birth to help calm their fears of birth.

Like *Aconite*, the woman who needs *Cimicifuga* or *Arsenicum* may also have a strong fear of death. The *Arsenicum* woman fears death for herself and is often also afraid for the health of her baby. The fear of *Aconite*, however, will be more extreme, sudden, and specific.

As with *Aconite*, the *Chamomilla* woman can also say

she wants to die and can't bear the pain. She is not anxious like *Aconite*, but is angry and impatient.

Arsenicum: This woman is anxious, restless and meticulous. She is not able to let go. Everything needs to be just right. She is a perfectionist and is very demanding. Her controlling personality stems from a fundamental insecurity about life. Her home is spotless and everything is in its place. She may spend her labor fanatically cleaning her house. Her vaginal muscles are very tight and it is difficult to do a vaginal exam because of this. Her second stage can be very long.

Every effort, however small, causes this woman to become greatly exhausted. She easily gets short of breath. Though she feels weak, there is great restlessness. This restlessness is due to her mental anxiety and fear. She fears death (although not as extreme as *Aconite's* fear of death). There is great anxiety and fearfulness for the health of the baby. She wants her partner to be with her constantly (see *Pulsatilla, Phosphorus*).

The *Arsenicum* woman is chilly, very sensitive to cold, and wants to be warmly wrapped up. Her mouth is dry and she is thirsty for frequent sips of cold water.

Belladonna: Suits the woman who is healthy, vital, and energetic. Everything seems intense. She is restless and in touch with her animal nature, uses strong primitive movements, loud noises, growling, or loud deep moaning. She does not want the support of others and prefers to solve problems on her own. Her extreme irritability causes her to become uncontrollably angry with the pains. She may explode in anger when you talk to her or try to help. Her imagination is vivid and can cause her to have visions and hallucinations. She seems to be in another world.

Her face is red and flushed. The pupils of her eyes are dilated. In extreme states, her eyes look wild and she may hit or bite. There is lots of heat, flushing, and congestion. Her face may be hot, but her extremities cold.

Everything happens suddenly. The contractions come and go suddenly, fly all over the place, may slow down, and sometimes stop. They are severe, sharp, cutting, shooting, come and go in repeated attacks and are painful but ineffective. She tends to push too early, causing her cervix to swell.

Bright lights, noise, and touch aggravate her, as well as any change to her circulation, such as becoming cold, overheated, or drafts. She is particularly aggravated by any jarring motion. A dark and quiet room is what she prefers. Her lips are chapped, her mouth is dry, but she is not thirsty and must be encouraged to drink during labor. She may, however, crave lemonade.

Caulophyllum: See above under "First Remedies to Consider."

Chamomilla: For extreme intolerance of pain (see *Coffea*). For failure to progress with extreme irritability.

This woman is angry and nasty due to over-sensitivity to pain. She is unable to bear even the slightest pain and says she can't or won't labor any longer. She snaps at you and curses. She will not permit a vaginal exam. Her cervix is rigid and can't stretch. Nothing you do pleases or helps her. She feels more should be done for her than is currently being done. You think she is well into active labor because of how much pain she seems to be experiencing, but, upon exam, her cervix is only 1 cm. dilated, or you feel the contractions and they are not very strong. She begs for pain relief or a cesarean section to end the pain and may even faint from it.

One cheek may be red and hot, the other pale and cold. The *Chamomilla* woman is thirsty, restless, hot, and wants to be uncovered.

The *Chamomilla* woman can look like *Cimicifuga*. *Cimicifuga* is hysterical and will scream, but is not as angry and cursing as *Chamomilla*. *Cimicifuga* tends to be more chilly.

Coffea also is highly sensitive to pain but is not irritable, angry, and harsh like *Chamomilla*.

Cimicifuga: See above under "First Remedies to Consider."

Coffea: For extreme sensitivity to pain (see *Chamomilla*). For the birthing woman who is highly sensitive, nervous, and overexcited.

The woman who *Coffea* would benefit is highly sensitive, nervous, and overexcited, similar to the state created by drinking too much coffee. She is extremely sensitive to pain; cannot bear even the slightest pain; complains, whines, cries out from the slightest pain (see *Chamomilla*). All her senses are very acute and oversensitive to any stimuli. She is sensitive to slight noise and odors, and adverse to being touched.

Her mind is very overexcited, with racing thoughts. She is very talkative, lively, gay, and ecstatic. On the other hand, she complains, is irritable, and nothing is right (see *Chamomilla*). This woman can go from excitable and restless to despairing and afraid of death; from talkativeness to moaning, screaming, and crying.

She us unable to sleep because of excitement, racing thoughts, and over-activity of the mind. The slightest noise wakes her. Her over-sensitivity can cause her to experience great fatigue and weakness. Any stimulation or strong emotion will aggravate her further.

With the *Coffea* woman, labor pains can be felt in the small of the back. The labor is ineffectual, the cervix doesn't dilate. Contractions are irregular, experienced as severe, and stop or slow down.

Coffea is similar to *Chamomilla* in their sensitivity to pain and irritability. The *Chamomilla* woman will tend to be more irritable, angry, snappish, rude, and harsh.

Giving a single dose of *Coffea* to a laboring woman who is overexcited and unable to relax or sleep will help her to relax and get the needed rest to continue with labor.

Gelsemium: Excellent remedy for dysfunctional labor with failure to progress. Excellent when there is fear of birth, given the day before or during labor. Used commonly to initiate labor.

The woman who needs *Gelsemium* is emotionally timid. She feels weak, very tired, and fearful in anticipation of labor and birth. Her fear is that she will not be able to persist and accomplish the birth. There will be generalized weakness with trembling, shivering, or nervous/emotional excitement (see *Caulophyllum, Cimicifuga, Opium*). Her legs especially will tremble nervously. She fears challenging tasks. She may chatter nervously during first stage.

Even before active labor begins, she feels weak and tired. There is inertia of the uterus. She looks drowsy and dull. Her eyes droop and her face is flushed. Her cervical os is rigid. The contractions start in the back and go to the abdomen. Labor pains are felt all in the back. The contractions may run down her legs or up her back. The pains are spasmodic. The contractions may cause the baby to ascend rather than descend. The contractions stop during vaginal exams because she is so nervous, and are weak from uterine inertia. Chills run up and down her back. She feels better after urination. She is typically chilly and thirstless.

When there is generalized fatigue and nervousness, or when *Caulophyllum* seems indicated for these symptoms but fails to act, *Gelsemium* is very likely to be effective. *Gelsemium* is thirstless, whereas *Caulophyllum* can be thirsty.

Gelsemium tends to be talkative like *Cimicifuga*. They both show nervous trembling. The *Gelsemium* woman's speech is very soft, slow, and almost slurred because of her general weakness and exhaustion.

Like *Gelsemium*, the *Aconite* state also has ailments from fright. The difference is that with the fright of *Aconite*, she experiences strong anxiety and heart palpitations. The anxiety comes and goes in waves. She tends to be thirsty for cold water, whereas those needing *Gelsemium* tend to be thirstless.

Gossypium: Excellent remedy to keep in mind for failure to progress in labor when the symptoms match.

The *Gossypium* woman's contractions tend to remain very weak, very mild, and almost painless no matter what is tried. She does not have to stop what she is doing during a contraction. The labor lingers and does not progress. Her cervical os is thick and rigid, and does not dilate. She is emotionally stable, but becomes extremely weak and tired from only a small number of contractions. There may be nausea from the weak contractions.

Ignatia: For failure to progress in labor associated with an emotional crisis. Any emotional crisis, particularly one of loss, grief, disappointment, or rejection can bring on the *Ignatia* state.

The typical *Ignatia* woman has high expectations and ideals have not been met by reality. The disappointment is unendurable. Her marriage may not be going well, a death may have occurred, or the birth may not be happening as she had hoped. She may be grieving the loss of the pregnancy and is having a hard time letting go.

She tries to keep her feelings inside because she doesn't want to be seen as emotionally weak, imperfect, or falling apart. She avoids breaking down in front of others (see *Natrum muriaticum*). This inner conflict leads to hysterical symptoms (see *Cimicifuga*). She becomes nervous and excitable. Her moods are very changeable and unpredictable. She has lots of mood swings. She avoids crying in front of others, but may break down into uncontrollable, hysterical sobbing, and often cries uncontrollably when she is alone. She does not like to be consoled or to admit that she has a problem. Because of her reluctance to show her real feelings, she may appear hard. She can be rude, insulting, critical, is often, in fact, self-critical, and is usually very sensitive to reprimand. You sense that something is going on underneath the surface. Her frequent sighing gives away her internal turmoil.

There is a lump in her throat and she tends to hold her breath. To breathe at all, she must take a deep breath (sigh). The tension of trying to hold her feelings in leads to spasmodic and erratic symptoms as well as cramps and spasms. There may be convulsive twitching of the muscles of her face or the corners of her mouth. Her contractions become weak or stop altogether. Her cervical os is rigid. She tends to be oversensitive to pain. Her limbs tend to tremble.

Think of *Ignatia* for a woman with a history of a deep grief after the birth of a previous child and whose current labor slows down or stops altogether. Maybe her previous baby was stillborn or she placed the baby for adoption. Her grief is suppressed. Unconsciously she does not want to let the birth take place because she fears losing this child also.

The differences between *Ignatia* and *Natrum muriaticum* need to be understood, as they are both remedies for grief that is held in. *Ignatia* is more useful for an acute or recent emotional crisis, whereas *Natrum muriaticum* is more for a chronic personality tendency. *Ignatia* tries to block out her feelings while *Natrum muriaticum* broods on them. The *Ignatia* woman will either sob hysterically with deep sighing or tense up and hold back from crying. The *Natrum muriaticum* type is more likely to talk about her feelings with tears running down her cheeks. She has a hard time letting go of and resolving grief, tending to hold on to it and to feel like nobody understands her.

The *Cimicifuga* state can look like *Ignatia* because of the hysterical tendency, the sighing, the crying, the negativity, and the ailments arising from grief. However, *Cimicifuga* is a more fragmented and dissociated state. The *Cimicifuga* type is more excitable and open, talking loquaciously about her complaints. *Ignatia* tends to be more reserved and does not show her deeper feelings as easily.

The following personal account illustrates the great benefit that *Ignatia* has to offer. I received a long distance call from Bev after the tragic stillbirths of her twin sons. The birth, besides being emotionally traumatic, had been physically very difficult for her. She was in a state of shock, keeping basically to herself, crying uncontrollably when alone, and unable to sleep at night. Though no remedy can do away with the pain of dealing with such a tragedy, *Ignatia* helped her to find inner strength, grieve more openly with her family and friends, ask for the support she needed, and to sleep at night. *Ignatia* would have helped Bev immensely during her difficult labor and delivery of the twins, though I was unfortunately not there to give it to her.

Two months went by and Bev called me again saying she was bleeding excessively and her physician wanted to give her medication to stop the bleeding. We talked about her grieving process and her tendency to keep her feelings locked up inside. She seemed angry and bitter about the loss of her sons. I mentioned that perhaps her womb was weeping its loss (the womb via bleeding is another outlet for tears in women). One dose of *Natrum muriaticum* high potency was given. Bev called me a few days later to report, much to her delight, that after passing a large blood clot, her bleeding had stopped almost completely within 24 hours of taking the remedy. More remarkable, however, was that the night of taking the remedy, she had dreamed about her sons for the first time since their death. They were doing fine in the spirit world and had sent her their love.

Read more about using *Ignatia* for an acute emotional crisis in the chapter "Healing From a Difficult

Delivery or Cesarean Section."

Natrum muriaticum: Excellent remedy for a cervix that does not dilate when the mental-emotional picture matches.

The *Natrum muriaticum* woman does not openly express her feelings. While being serious and often humorless, she is very sensitive and other's emotions affect her deeply. She gets hurt easily and closes off to prevent being hurt. During labor, she becomes depressed, withdrawn, wants to be alone, doesn't ask for anything, and becomes difficult to reach. Though she may be very sad, her feelings are held inside and she will not cry. A previous grief, i.e., miscarriage, stillbirth, cesarean, etc., may have been suffered and is being kept inside (see *Ignatia*). She is much worse if you try and console her, preferring to cry alone. Showing her intimate feelings is embarrassing to her.

This type of woman does not open up, and so her cervix does not open up. Her pushing stage is very long because she cannot open up. In order for labor to progress, she must take her mind off of things.

Labor pains will be slow, stopping or slowing down, and are weak. Often, there is exhaustion, even if the labor has just started. The contractions may stop if anyone comes into the room. She tends to be thirsty. It is impossible for her to urinate in front of others.

Nux vomica: For failure to progress in labor when with every contraction there is an urge to move her bowels or urinate, but only a small amount or nothing is passed. This urge is not due to the pressure of the baby's head, which is normal during transition and second stage.

The *Nux vomica* woman tends to be high-strung and irritable. She is impatient, very easily angered or offended, does not like to be contradicted, and can be abusive.

The contractions may be very spasmodic and severe, and suddenly cease entirely. She is hypersensitive to pain (see *Chamomilla, Coffea*). The labor pains can cause her to faint. Also there is sensitivity to odors, noise, light, and all external stimuli. She tends to be chilly.

Opium: Failure to progress with great fear (see *Aconite, Gelsemium*) and painlessness. This remedy is unfortunately no longer legally available in the U.S. due to the F.D.A. It is an important remedy, however, so I have included it here. It is totally safe in homeopathic form.

The woman who would benefit from *Opium* has deep fears that are partially expressed or are suppressed into a stuporous, sleepy state. Think of it if the mother is excessively sleepy during labor and experiences no pain where it normally would exist. She may be frightened to go into labor, because of the intensity of the contractions, or by what she *thinks* are excessive movements of the baby (see *Gelsemium*). The contractions become very mild or stop because of the fright. She is withdrawn and disconnected from her feelings and the outer world, says there is no problem, and does not understand why her body is not responding. There is a far away, hazy look in her eyes. She is in a euphoric, peaceful, drowsy, dreamlike state, and may alternate between stupor and restlessness. Because of her withdrawn state, she does not bond with her newborn (see *Sepia*).

The woman needing *Opium* is often constipated in the beginning of labor when normally there is increased bowel activity. This is because of her deep fear. She is very warm-blooded, aggravated by heat, and has hot perspiration. The bed may feel so hot, that she cannot lie in it. Her breathing is often heavy, labored, and noisy. Her face may be puffy and flushed deep red or mottled purple. Her muscles can twitch, tremble, and jerk, especially her face muscles. Her limbs tremble from fright (see *Gelsemium*).

The *Gelsemium* and *Aconite* types both have fear of labor and birth. *Gelsemium* is timid, weak, and tired, whereas *Opium* is more sleepy and dreamlike. *Gelsemium* is chilly and thirstless. *Opium* is very hot.

Aconite's fear is more intense and specific. She *knows* she is going to die. With the fright she experiences strong anxiety and heart palpitations. She tends to be very thirsty for cold water.

The *Sepia* woman is withdrawn and irritable because she is worn-out and at the end of her rope. *Opium* is withdrawn into a euphoric, dreamlike, nonresponsive state. *Sepia* is chilly, sensitive to cold, and likes to be covered up warmly. *Opium* is very warm-blooded and aggravated by heat.

Think of *Opium* for newborn asphyxia if the mother has been in an *Opium* state. Also think of it for a premature delivery from fear or fright.

Phosphorus: Think of *Phosphorus* for the woman who is very open, sensitive, intuitive, and impressionable. Her captivating quality is expressive, spontaneous, and easily connects with others. She is emotionally open, trusting, sympathetic, and wants to communicate and to have others near by. She loves massage, physical contact, closeness with others, and is often very spiritually aware.

Her openness and imagination lack boundaries, so she is very suggestible and excitable. This causes her to easily experience the same feelings as someone else, even to the point of being clairvoyant. She may be very ungrounded, dreamy, and spaced out (see *Opium*). Many fears and anxieties are experienced, especially at night or when alone. She startles easily and is afraid of being alone, the dark, thunderstorms, death, robbers, disease, and that something bad will happen. There may be a fear that something will go wrong with the baby. She may fear childbirth and that she will have to have a cesarean. She is dependent on her birth attendant. The reassurance of others is important to her and she is easily reassured. Talking helps her to feel better.

Her labor pains can be distressing and nonproductive. There may be a sense of weakness and emptiness in her abdomen.

The woman who *Phosphorus* benefits can be tall, thin, delicate, fine featured and long fingered. Often her hair is reddish. Her energy burns out quickly. There is a tendency to easy bruising and bleeding, i.e., nosebleeds and hemorrhaging, so be prepared to give her a dose postpartum, if needed. She may have developed a blue discoloration of her face during pregnancy.

Along with being very thirsty for ice cold drinks and sodas, she loves ice cream, chocolate, salty, and spicy foods. Her metabolism is fast. She feels better and more grounded from eating. She may vomit after drinking cold drinks when they become warm in her stomach.

The *Phosphorus* woman may be confused with

Arsenicum because of the anxiety and weakness. *Phosphorus* is easily reassured because of her suggestibility. *Arsenicum* is more controlling and demanding. *Phosphorus* is thirsty for large amounts of ice cold drinks, while *Arsenicum's* thirst is for frequent sips.

The *Pulsatilla* type is also open, afraid of being alone, and afraid of the dark. She tends to be more changeable, timid, tearful, and needy than *Phosphorus*. *Pulsatilla* has no thirst, and *Phosphorus* is very thirsty. *Pulsatilla* tends to be more warm blooded and aggravated by heat. *Pulsatilla* is a more commonly prescribed remedy for pregnancy and birth.

The fearfulness of *Phosphorus* may remind you of other fearful remedies, but the personality features of *Phosphorus* are quite distinct and characteristic.

Platina: Extreme sensitiveness of the vagina, cervical os, and pudendum (external genitalia). The sensitiveness is so extreme that the *Platina* woman is unable to concentrate on labor. She cannot bear for anything to touch her genitalia and cannot bear to be examined. Her contractions are weak, spasmodic, painful, but ineffectual. The pains reach a certain point, then cease. They may be all felt on the left-side.

She is haughty, takes control, and looks down on everyone. Her passionate nature is dramatic, talkative, and paranoid. Her dark thoughts cause her great anxiety. A high sexual desire is often experienced.

Pulsatilla: The use of this remedy is generally based on the mental-emotional state.

The woman who *Pulsatilla* would benefit is focused on how she feels about things. Her emotions are very much on the surface. The tears flow easily and she feels much better from crying. Her nature is generally soft, loving, and affectionate, but can be irritable also. Her moods are very changeable. There is a strong need for affection, attention, and reassurance from others. This type woman relies on others for her emotional well-being, feels easily forsaken and miserable, but is easily reassured. She may ask her partner often if he loves her. Conflicts are avoided because of her desire for harmony. She is very obedient to her birth attendant. Because she thinks she isn't doing a good job, there will be tears. She keeps apologizing, especially about inconveniencing others. She needs lots of reassurance, feels vulnerable, and does not want to be left alone. Her husband/partner won't be allowed to leave her side for any reason. The more people she has around her, caring for her, the more energy she has.

Changeability is a strong symptom of *Pulsatilla*. There is changeability on all levels. She has emotional highs and lows throughout labor. Even the physical pain is changeable. The labor tries to get going, the contractions come and go, but labor never gets established; or labor seems to be happening nicely, but no progress is made.

The contractions may be felt in the back, be short, irregular, weak, slow down or completely stop. She feels faint and suffocated with the contractions, and may have heart palpitations. She may actually faint during difficult labor.

The *Pulsatilla* woman has a strong desire for open air and must have the windows open with the contractions. She gets warm quickly and is intolerant of heat. Though usually warm-blooded, she can be chilly. Even though her lips and mouth may be dry, she is relatively thirstless. She may drink to cool herself down. Rich and fatty foods aggravate her. She always feels worse from heat , better from open air, and typically blushes easily.

Pulsatilla is useful at any time during labor, birth or postpartum when this mental-emotional state is seen.

Secale: *Secale* is especially indicated for elderly women or for women who have had a number of children close together (see *Sepia*). (Note: "Elderly" is a term used in the old homeopathic books and by modern obstetrics, usually referring to a woman of 35 years of age or older who is assumed to have poor uterine tone. This lack of uterine tone can be seen in women who have had more than one child, particularly those who have had a number of children close together. Not all women who are 35 years or older, however, fit this description. Each woman should be assessed individually for her overall level of health and vitality regardless of her age.)

The woman who *Secale* would benefit has contractions that are weak or absent because her uterus has no tone. She tends to be thin and feels weak and exhausted. Everything seems too loose and too open. She has prolonged bearing down sensations, but the contractions are irregular. Labor lingers and no progress is made in dilation. The contractions may be strong for a short period of time, but still there is no progress. *Secale* can strengthen the uterus so it will work effectively.

Emotionally this woman tends to be timid, shy, quiet, and lack self confidence. She can also be fearful and suspicious.

Secale, unlike *Sepia*, is usually burning hot and cannot tolerate covers, though her skin may be cold to the touch. She feels better from open air, being fanned, cold, and from uncovering.

She may experience tingling all over her skin. She likes to be rubbed and massaged lightly. She may also have the strange symptom of being very bothered if her fingers touch each other. She must hold her fingers spread apart.

Sepia: With *Sepia* we think of someone who is worn out and at the end of her rope. This may be from trying to do too much in her life or from the demands of too many children (see *Secale*). This pregnancy may not have been wanted.

The *Sepia* woman is very tired, wants to be left alone, and not be bothered. However, she dreads being completely alone. Consolation is disagreeable to her. She is very critical, easily irritated by small things, and often makes sarcastic, cutting remarks. She feels indifferent and detached from her husband/partner and family. In extreme cases, there is anger and hatred towards the baby with a desire to hurt the child. These feelings may scare and horrify her. Her state of mind can cause her great guilt.

Sepia is often sad, depressed, and feels like there is a black cloud hanging over her (see *Cimicifuga*). There may be involuntary weeping without knowing why (see *Pulsatilla*).

Her pelvis feels congested with a sensation of heaviness. There is a strong bearing down sensation. The *Sepia* woman feels as if the baby will fall out of her vagina and may cross her legs to keep this from happening. There may be a sense of weight in her anus like a heavy ball, due to the laxness of her tissues. This sensation, though not due to the pressure of the baby's head, may make her want to push regardless. The contractions are spasmodic and irregular. She has fine darting pains in the cervix from below upward and may feel better from drawing up her legs. Her cervical os is rigid and tight.

This woman is chilly, has cold hands and feet, is sensitive to the cold, and has flushes of heat. She likes being covered up warmly (opposite of *Secale*). Vigorous motion, especially dancing, causes her to feel better, but she may be afraid the baby will fall out. There may be yellow or brown spots on her face (chloasma) or a yellow saddle across her nose. She is usually thin, but not always. She tends to be constipated.

Sepia is an excellent remedy for the prevention and treatment of uterine prolapse. It is also excellent for postpartum depression for the woman who feels detached from, or may even hate, her baby and husband/partner.

Repertory for Prolonged, Difficult, or Dysfunctional Labor

A repertory is made up of rubrics and sub-rubrics. A rubric is a symptom of homeopathic significance followed by the main remedies that cover that symptom. Each rubric (symptom) may be broken down into finer levels of detail, called sub-rubrics. These sub-rubrics are indented under a main rubric so you know that they relate to the bigger one. There may be several levels of indentation. Rubrics, sub-rubrics, and remedies are listed alphabetically. See the remedy index at the back of the book for remedy abbreviations. Remedies are graded as **Bold**, <u>Underline</u>, or Plain. **Bold** means that the symptom is very strong and distinct for that remedy. <u>Underline</u> means that symptom is strong for that remedy. Plain means that symptom is present for that remedy. When only one remedy in plain type is shown for a symptom, that remedy is the main one to consider for that symptom.

PROLONGED, DIFFICULT, OR DYSFUNCTIONAL LABOR: *Acon., Ars., Bell., Caul., Cimic., Cham., Coff., Gels., Goss., Ign., Nat-m., Nux-v., Op., Phos., Plat., Puls., Sec., Sep.*
Arn., Carbo-v., Kali-c. are written about in other chapters. Check the "Remedy Index" in back of the book.

FAILURE TO PROGRESS (dilation of cervical os slow): Could be any of the remedies above. Also see "Rigidity of cervical os" below. First remedies to consider: Caul., Cimic.

FETAL HEART RATE, to improve during pushing
stage: Carb-v.

GENERAL SYMPTOMS:
Air, desire for open: Acon., **Puls.**, <u>Sec.</u>
Body temperature: (Most pregnant women are
commonly warm. Use body temperature
only to differentiate between two or more
remedies if her body temperature is intense
or unusual.)
Chilly: **Acon., Ars.,** <u>Caul., Cimic., Gels.,</u>
Ign., <u>Nat-m.,</u> **Nux-v., Phos., Plat., Puls.,**
<u>Sep.</u>
Hot: <u>Cham.,</u> **Coff., Nat-m.,** <u>Nux-v., Op.,</u>
<u>Phos.,</u> **Puls., Sec.**
Exhaustion: See chapter, "Routinely Useful
Birth Remedies" for remedies for general
exhaustion.
Causing contractions to be weak or slow
down: Arn., <u>Caul.,</u> Gels., Goss., Nat-m.,
Sec., Sep.
Long and exhausting labor and birth,
from a: Arn., Carbo-v., Caul.
Depleted to the point of collapse:
Carbo-v.
Uterine atony (lack of tone), from, in
women who have had many
children close together: Sec., Sep.
Air, desire for open: Sec.
Chilly and desires to be covered: Sep.
Hot and cannot tolerate being
covered: Sec.
Effort, after every little, with nervous
restlessness, anxiety, and a need to have
everything in control: Ars.
Emotional suppression, with: Nat-m.
Labor almost painless: Goss.

Exhaustion (continued):
    Motion, better from vigorous (dancing):
        Sep.
    Timidity and nervousness, with: Gels.
Fainting: <u>Acon.</u>, Arn., <u>Ars.</u>, Bell., <u>Cham.</u>, <u>Cimic.</u>,
    <u>Coff.</u>, <u>Ign.</u>, **Nux-v.**, **Puls.**, **Sec.**, <u>Sep.</u>
    From an acute emotional crisis: Ign.
    From sensitiveness to pain: Cham.
Sensitive:
    Noise, to: Bell., Cimic., <u>Coff.</u>, <u>Ign.</u>, Nux-v.
    Pain, to: Acon., Arn., **Bell.**, **Cham.**, Cimic.,
        Coff., **Ign.**, **Nux-v.**, <u>Phos.</u>, Puls., <u>Sec.</u>,
        Sep.
        Bruised and sore, feels: <u>Arn.</u>
        Die, with certainty she will: **Acon.**
        Emotional crisis, from an acute: Ign.
        Fainting from: Cham. (See "Fainting"
            above.)
        Intolerable, pains are: **Cham.**, Cimic.,
            Coff.
        Desperate, make her: <u>Cham.</u>
        Irritability, with extreme: **Cham.**
        Nervous sensitivity and excitability,
            with: **Coff.**
    Vagina, oversensitive, interrupting labor
        pains: <u>Plat.</u>
Sleeplessness: <u>Coff.</u>
Sleepy (drowsy): Gels., **Op.**, <u>Puls.</u>
    After each contraction: Gels.
Thirst, unquenchable: <u>Acon.</u>, **Ars.**, Cham.,
    <u>Nat-m.</u>, **Phos.**
    For large, quantities of ice cold drinks: Phos.
    For small sips, often: Ars.
Thirstless: <u>Bell.</u>, **Gels.**, <u>Kali-c.</u>, <u>Op.</u>, **Puls.**, <u>Sep.</u>
Trembling: Caul., Cimic., Gels., Ign.
    Emotional crisis, from an acute: Ign.

Trembling (continued):
    Hysteria, with: Cimic., Gels.
    Nervousness, from: Cimic., Gels.
    Weakness, from: Caul., Gels.

LABOR PAINS (contractions):
    Alternate with hemorrhage: **Puls.**
    Amniotic fluid gone, with: Bell.
    Bearing down pains: Bell., Sec., Sep.
        Better crossing her legs: Sep.
        Feels as if the baby would fall out: Sep.
    Changeable: **Puls.**
    Child seems to ascend with each contraction:
        <u>**Gels.**</u>
    Darting upward from cervix: Sep.
    Desperate, make her: <u>Cham.</u>
    Extending to back: Cham., Gels., Kali-c.
    Extending to hips: Cimic., Gels.
    Extending into thighs: Cham., <u>Kali-c.</u>
    Extending upward: **Cham.**, Gels., Puls.
    Fainting, cause: <u>Cimic.</u>, **Nux-v.**, <u>Puls.</u> (See
        "Fainting" above.)
        From sensitiveness to pain: Cham.
    Hourglass contractions: Bell., Cham., <u>Kali-c.</u>,
        Nux-v., <u>Plat.</u>, Puls., Sec., <u>Sep.</u>
    Ineffectual: Acon., Arn., Bell., Caul., Cham.,
        Cimic., <u>Coff.</u>, Gels., **Kali-c.**, Nux-v., Op.,
        Phos., Plat., **Puls.**, Sec., Sep.
    Intermittent: **Caul.**
    Irregular: Arn., <u>Caul.</u>, Cham., Cimic., <u>Coff.</u>,
        Nux-v., **Puls.**, Sec.
    Left-sided: **Plat.**
    Needle, like a: Caul., Sep.
    Open and loose, everything seems, without
        action: Sec.

Labor pains (continued):
  Painful, feel too: Acon., Arn., **Bell.**, **Cham.**,
      Cimic., **Coff.**, **Nux-v.**, <u>Phos.</u>, Puls., <u>Sec.</u>, **Sep.**
    Bruised and sore, feels: <u>Arn.</u>
    Die, with certainty she will: **Acon.**
    Intolerable, pains are: **Cham.**, **Coff.**
      Desperate, make her: <u>Cham.</u>
      Irritability, with extreme: **Cham.**
      Nervous sensitivity and excitability,
        with: **Coff.**
  Painless, almost: <u>Goss.</u>, <u>Op.</u>
  Presentation abnormal: Puls.
  Short: <u>Caul.</u>, <u>Puls.</u>
  Slowing down: Arn., **Bell.**, <u>Caul.</u>, <u>Cham.</u>,
      Cimic., <u>Coff.</u>, Gels., Ign., **Kali-c.**, <u>Nat-m.</u>,
      <u>Nux-v.</u>, **Op.**, Phos., Plat., **Puls.**, **Sec.**, <u>Sep.</u>
    Cramps in hips, from: Cimic.
    Emotional crisis, from an acute: Ign.
    Emotional excitement, from: Cimic., Gels.
    Emotional suppression, from: Ign., Nat-m.
    Exhaustion, from a long and exhausting
      labor: Arn., Carbo-v., Caul.
      Depleted to the point of collapse:
        Carbo-v.
    Fright, from: Acon.
    Nervous trembling, with: Caul., Cimic.,
      Gels., Ign.
    Uterine atony (lack of tone), from, in
      women who have had a number of
      children close together: Sec., Sep.
      Air, desire for open: Sec.
      Chilly and desires to be covered: Sep.
      Hot and cannot tolerate being covered:
        Sec.
  Spasmodic: Arn., <u>Bell.</u>, **Caul.**, **Cham.**, <u>Cimic.</u>,
      Coff., **Gels.**, Ign., Kali-c., <u>Nux-v.</u>, <u>Op.</u>, Phos.,
      Plat., **Puls.**, <u>Sec.</u>, <u>Sep.</u>

Labor pains (continued):

Stool, causing urging to: **Nux-v.**, Plat.

Stop, suppressed, or wanting: Acon., Arn.,
Caul., Cimic., Gels., Ign., Nat-m., Nux-v.,
Op., Plat., Puls., Sec.

Emotional crisis, from an acute: Ign.

Emotional suppression, from: Ign., Nat-m.

Exhaustion, from a long and exhausting
labor: Arn., Carbo-v., Caul.

Depleted to the point of collapse:
Carbo-v.

Fear, from: Op.

Grief or fear, from a past suppressed:
Cimic., Ign.

Stopping suddenly and convulsions and
coma set in: Op.

Uterine atony (lack of tone), from, in
women who have had a number of
children close together: Sec., Sep.

Air, desire for open: Sec.

Chilly and desires to be covered: Sep.

Hot and cannot tolerate being
covered: Sec.

Strong, too (violent): Acon., **Arn.**, Bell., Caul.,
Cham., Coff., Nux-v., Phos., Plat., Sec., Sep.

Sudden: Bell.

Uncoordinated: See "Spasmodic" above.

Weak: Arn., Bell., Caul., Cham., **Cimic.**, Coff.,
Gels., Goss., Ign., **Kali-c.**, **Nat-m.**, Nux-v.,
Op., Phos., Plat., **Puls.**, Sec., Sep. (See
"Labor pains, Slowing down" above.)

MENTAL AND EMOTIONAL SYMPTOMS:

Anger/rage: Bell., **Cham.**, Nux-v.

Towards the baby, which horrify her: Sep.

Anxiety: See "Fear/Anxiety" below.

Mental and emotional symptoms (continued):
    Aversion, to her husband/partner and family:
        <u>Sep.</u>
    Bond, does not, with baby: Op., Sep.
        With irritability: Sep.
        Nonresponsive, dreamlike state: Op.
    Bossy (dictatorial): Ars., Plat.
    Company:
        Aversion to: Cham., Sep.
        Desire for, cannot be alone: Ars., Bell.,
            Kali-c., **Phos.**, <u>Puls.</u>
    Complaining: Cimic., Cham., Coff., Ign., Nux-v.
    Control, need to have everything in, with
        nervous restlessness and anxiety: Ars.
    Crisis, acute emotional: Ign.
    Die, sure that she will: Acon.
    Dream, as if in a: Op., Phos.
    Emotions suppressed: Ign., Nat-m. (See "Grief"
        below.)
    Fear/Anxiety:
        Labor, during: Acon., Ars., Cimic., Coff.,
            Nat-m., Op., Phos., Plat.
            Control, need to have everything in:
                Ars.
            Death of: Ars., **Acon.**, Cimic., <u>Coff.,</u> Plat.
            Sure that she will die: **Acon.**
            Control, need to have everything in,
                with nervous restlessness and
                anxiety: Ars.
            Disabling fear from past unbearably
                painful memory: Cimic.
            Reassured easily (consolation
                ameliorates): <u>Phos</u>, **Puls.**
            Suppressed into dreamlike, sleepy state:
                Op.
            Transition, during: Acon.
         Labor, of: **Gels.**, Kali-c.

Mental and emotional symptoms (continued):
    Fragmented: Cimic., Ign.
    Grief: Cimic., Ign., Nat-m.
        Acute emotional crisis: Ign.
        Prefers to grieve alone: **Ign., Nat-m.**
    Haughty: Acon., Arn., Ars., Bell., Ign., Nat-m.,
        Nux-v., Phos., **Plat.**, <u>Puls.</u>, Sec.
        Delusion of superiority: <u>Plat.</u>
    Hysteria: **Gels., Cimic.**, Ign.
    Idealistic: <u>Ign.</u>, <u>Plat.</u>
    Impressionable: Coff., <u>Phos.</u>, <u>Puls.</u>
    Mood changeable (moody): <u>Ign.</u>, **Puls.**
    Perfectionist: **Ars.**, Ign.
    Sadness: Cimic., <u>Ign.</u>, Nat-m., Puls., Sep.
        With an acute emotional crisis: Ign.
        With weariness and exhaustion: <u>Sep.</u>
    Screaming (shrieking), with the pain: **Acon.,**
        <u>Bell.</u>, **Cham., Coff.**
    Sighing: <u>Cimic.</u>, **Ign.**
    Soft and sweet (yielding): Caul., **Puls.**
    Timid: **Gels., Puls.**, Sec.
    Weeping: <u>Coff.</u>, Ign., Plat., **Puls.**, Sep.
        Delivered, because she has not, with intense
            uterine inertia: <u>Puls.</u>
        Difficulty weeping: Nat-m.
        Feels much better from: Puls.
        Hysterically, from acute emotional crisis:
            Ign.
        Uncontrollable weeping from grief: Ign.
        Wants to be alone to weep: Ign., <u>Nat-m.</u>

RIGIDITY:
    Cervical os, of: Acon., <u>Bell.</u>, **Caul., Cham.,**
        Cimic., Gels., Ign., Nux-v., Sec.
    Vagina, of: Ars.

URGING (desire), to move her bowels or urinate with each contraction: **Nux-v.**, Plat.

VAGINAL EXAMS:
>   Difficult to do because her vaginal muscles are very tight: Ars.
>   Intolerant of:
>>   Fear, with extreme: Acon.
>>   Touching her genitalia, cannot bear anything, because the sensitiveness is so extreme: Plat.

CHAPTER 8

Back Labor and Posterior Position of the Baby

A posterior position is when the baby is head down, but with her back along the mother's back (facing the mother's front instead of her back). Though this is a normal position for the baby, with most babies turning sometime during labor, it can slow down labor or completely arrest it. Some labors can get stuck in late first or early second stage, as the baby's head undergoes back-to-front rotation, and further molding is required to allow it to slip under the pubic bone and be born. In a small percentage of cases this anterior rotation never occurs and the baby is born "sunny-side-up," if the mom's pelvis is large enough. Posterior labors and births are more difficult for mom and baby because a wider diameter of the baby's head must pass through the pelvis. It tends to cause strong back pains during contractions.

Being in a hands and knees position during labor uses gravity to help turn a posterior baby. Also have the birthing woman try pelvic rocking between contractions while in a hands and knees position. Gently massaging her belly in the direction you want the baby to move in encourages the baby to turn. If you are sure of which side the baby's back is on, have the laboring woman lie on the opposite side. Again, this uses gravity.

Remedies to Consider:

Belladonna: Suits a healthy, vital, and energetic woman. Everything seems intense. She is irritable, restless, and in touch with her animal nature. Her back feels as if it will break.

Read more about *Belladonna* in the chapter "Prolonged, Difficult, or Dysfunctional Labor."

Caulophyllum: When labor is stalled because of a posterior position of the baby and no other remedy is indicated, try *Caulophyllum* 200c every hour for a few hours. Word of caution: *Caulophyllum* will bring on strong contractions, so don't use it if the contractions are already very forceful.

Chamomilla: For back labor from a posterior baby with extreme sensitivity to pain.

This woman is angry and nasty due to over-sensitivity to pain. She is unable to bear even the slightest pain. Her back feels like it is splitting apart. She can't bear any touch or examination because she is too sensitive.

Read more about *Chamomilla* in the chapter "Prolonged, Difficult, or Dysfunctional Labor."

Coffea: For the birthing woman who is highly sensitive, nervous, and overexcited.

The woman who needs *Coffea* is extremely sensitive to pain; cannot bear even the slightest pain;

complains, whines, and cries out (see *Chamomilla*). All her senses are very acute and oversensitive to any stimuli. Her labor pains can be felt in the small of the back. The labor is ineffectual and the cervix doesn't dilate. The contractions are irregular, experienced as severe, and slow down, or stop.

Read more about *Coffea* in the chapter "Prolonged, Difficult, or Dysfunctional Labor."

Gelsemium: Excellent remedy for back labor and failure to progress (possibly from a posterior position of the baby).

This birthing woman feels weak, very tired, and fearful. There typically will be generalized weakness with trembling, shivering, or nervous/emotional excitement. Her legs especially will tremble nervously. She fears that she will not be able to persist and accomplish the birth.

The labor pains are felt all in the back . They start in the back and go to the abdomen. Contractions may run down her legs or up her back. Her cervical os is rigid. The contractions are spasmodic and can cause the baby to ascend rather than descend. They (contractions) can be weak from uterine inertia and fear. During vaginal exams, contractions stop because she is so nervous. She is typically chilly and thirstless.

Read more about *Gelsemium* in the chapter "Prolonged, Difficult, or Dysfunctional Labor."

Kali carbonicum: For back labor (possibly from a posterior position of the baby) with a nagging lower backache that may extend to the buttocks. She wants constant vigorous rubbing or hard pressure on her lower back, which somewhat relieves the pain. For stalled or arrested labors due to difficulty of anterior rotation of the fetal head with these symptoms.

Sharp, stitching pains stay in the lumbar region of the back. The uterine pains are hardly even there. She walks or sits with her hand held firmly against her lower back or will beg for someone to apply hard pressure on her lower back during contractions. Repeat the remedy if the symptoms relapse.

Nux vomica: For back labor that extends to the buttocks and thighs. With every contraction the *Nux vomica* woman feels she has to move her bowels or urinate, but only a small amount or nothing is passed. This urge is not due to the pressure of the baby's head, which is normal during transition and second stage.

She tends to be high-strung, irritable, impatient, and very easily angered or offended. She does not like to be contradicted and can be abusive.

The back pain is similar to that of *Kali carbonicum*, but *Nux vomica* will *not* want any pressure on her back. The pain is worse from pressure.

Pulsatilla: Think of *Pulsatilla* for the woman who has a strong need for affection, attention, approval, and reassurance from others. Her emotions are on the surface. She is easily moved to tears and feels much better from crying. She tends to be soft, sweet, affectionate, and sympathetic. She wants plenty of fresh air and will probably have the windows wide open.

Read more about *Pulsatilla* in the chapter "Prolonged, Difficult, or Dysfunctional Labor."

Sepia: *Sepia* can have back pain that comes on suddenly and is spasmodic. This woman can have frequent bearing down pains in her back and abdomen. Her back pain is better from hard pressure (see *Kali carbonicum*). She is tired, worn out, irritable, and wants to be left alone.

Read more about *Sepia* in the chapter "Prolonged, Difficult, or Dysfunctional Labor."

Repertory for Back Labor and Posterior Position of the Baby

(An explanation of repertory structure and remedy grading can be found in the beginning of the "Repertory For Prolonged, Difficult, or Dysfunctional Labor," page 61. See the remedy index at the back of the book for remedy abbreviations.)

BACK, LABOR PAINS FELT IN: *Bell., Caul., Cham., Coff., Gels., Kali-c., Nux-v., Puls., Sep.*
  Bearing down pains: Sep.
  Break or split apart, feels as if her back would: Bell., Cham.
  Contractions weak: Caul.
  Mood changeable (moody): **Puls.**
  Pain ascends during labor: **Gels.**
  Pain descends during labor: <u>Nux-v.</u>
  Pressure, better from hard: **Kali-c., Sep.**
  Pressure, worse from: Cham., Nux-v.
  Sensitive, pains are intolerable: **Cham., Coff.**
    Desperate, make her: <u>Cham.</u>
    Irritability, with extreme: **Cham.**
    Nervous sensitivity and excitability, with: **Coff.**
  Soft and sweet (yielding): **Puls.**
  Sudden and spasmodic (paroxysmal): Bell., Cham., Kali-c., <u>Nux-v., Sep.</u>
    Break, feels as if her back would: Bell.
    Pressure, better from hard: **Kali-c., Sep.**
    Pressure, worse from: Nux-v.
    Sensitivity, extreme to pain: Cham.
  Through to, and up the back: <u>Gels.</u>
  Timid and with exhaustion: Gels.
  Urging (desire), to move her bowels or urinate with each contraction: **Nux-v.**

CHAPTER 9

Routinely Useful Birth Remedies

Arnica montana: *Arnica* has been used for centuries to promote rapid healing. Use it routinely, giving a high potency dose (200c or whatever you have on hand) during labor, and another dose right after birth.

Arnica is miraculous in its ability to promote healing, control bleeding, prevent and reduce swelling and bruising, prevent tearing, shock, and infections, help the uterus to contract and expel the placenta, and relieve the sore, bruised feeling common after birth.

Arnica also helps with fatigue during labor, especially when the birthing woman feels sore, bruised, and exhausted. Give an occasional 30c dose for this purpose.

Kali phosphoricum: Can be used routinely for simple physical exhaustion during labor when there are no other symptoms or too few to prescribe another remedy. Give a 6x between every contraction for up to 6 doses until the energy level rises.

Rescue Remedy: A combination of five of Edward Bach's flower remedies. It is a wonderful all-purpose remedy, though not strictly homeopathic. *Rescue Remedy* was formulated as an emergency medicine. It is very calming and is useful for any type of emotional or physical distress, shock, panic, or fear. It can also be used for tiredness during labor. Use it on its own merit or if you are not sure what homeopathic remedy is indicated.

Put a few drops of the tincture in a cup of pure water and have the birthing woman sip as needed. It can be taken once for a minor injury or distress, or up to every few minutes in a serious situation. It can also be added to a bath (about 7 drops) for a relaxing and healing soak.

CHAPTER *10*

Routinely Useful Postpartum Remedies

Arnica montana: The most generally useful postpartum remedy. *Arnica* will promote healing, control bleeding, prevent tearing, reduce swelling and bruising, prevent shock and infections, help the uterus contract and expel the placenta, and relieve the sore, bruised feeling common after birth. It will also help to prevent or relieve afterpains.

Use it routinely in labor, when another remedy is not required, giving a high potency dose (200c or whatever you have on hand) during labor and another dose right after birth.

It is particularly indicated when the woman feels sore and bruised, in one area of her body or all over. The bed feels too hard. She is restless, cannot find a comfortable position, and does not want to be touched or approached because of the soreness. This woman often, though not always, is irritable and wants to be left alone. She says there is nothing the matter with her when you know there is.

Bellis perennis: For bruised soreness specifically of the abdominal wall and pelvic organs after childbirth, where *Arnica* has either not helped or has stopped helping, use *Bellis perennis*. It is particularly useful for multips with weak abdominal muscles. The uterus feels sore, as if squeezed. (Note: A multip refers to a woman who has already birthed one child.)

CHAPTER 11

Postpartum Hemorrhage

A certain amount of bleeding postpartum is normal, but bleeding must be closely monitored and managed in order to avoid a potential hemorrhage. A postpartum hemorrhage is an emergency situation and demands immediate emergency management from the birth attendant. It is defined as more than 2 cups of bleeding following birth. This could be from a small, constant trickle to a fast, profuse bleed, or anything in between. Don't wait for this much bleeding to occur before acting. *Act immediately to control bleeding.* Determining the cause of the bleeding will help you to know how to respond and deal with the situation effectively. Stay calm, put the baby to the breast to nurse (unless the situation is severe), have the new mom visualize her uterus contracting, and proceed with the following:

Though the cause of bleeding may be due to a partially separated placenta or cervical tear, these are very rare, assuming the birth has been well managed. Do not massage or otherwise handle the uterus before the placenta completely separates on its own, as this can cause severe hemorrhaging. A vaginal tear may also cause excessive bleeding and should be checked for and dealt with. This again is not common. The usual cause of postpartum bleeding is an atonic uterus, a uterus that does not contract well for a number of possible reasons, such as being overexhausted or having a full bladder.

Be sure to have the laboring woman urinate and fully empty her bladder prior to birthing her baby. Do this even if she does not have the urge. It is easy with all the intense sensations that she is experiencing to be numb to this basic sensation. A full bladder does not allow the uterus to fully contract, thus leading to a possible hemorrhage after the baby is born. A full bladder will cause the uterus to lie towards the right side of the pelvis instead of in the middle. You can also usually see it bulging out abdominally above her pubic bone. If this is the case, have her urinate into a bed pan or onto some towels without moving out of bed, and you should see an immediate improvement.

Do your best during labor to prevent the birthing woman from becoming overexhausted. An overexhausted woman has an overexhausted uterus that will not contract properly, leading to a possible hemorrhage. Preventing exhaustion involves making sure she is well rested and nourished *before* going into labor, keeping her environment stress-free during labor, helping her be as relaxed as possible, with her dozing off between contractions, and making changes if her labor stalls for too long. (Note: Read more about managing labor in the chapter "Prolonged, Difficult, or Dysfunctional Labor.")

After the placenta is delivered, check the uterus to make sure it is well-contracted. It should be felt in the middle, with the fundus (top of the uterus) slightly above, at, or below the umbilicus, be very firm, and about the size of a grapefruit. Putting the baby to the breast to nurse will cause strong contractions, thus preventing excess bleeding.

If there is slow continuous bleeding or spurts of blood, firmly massage the top of the uterus until it is well contracted. Apply downward pressure while firmly massaging *and* protecting the uterus from prolapsing with your other hand abdominally bracing the uterus upwards. This will expel any clots and membranes that might be left in the uterus and causing the bleeding. Keep massaging the uterus until it is well-contracted and again anytime bleeding reoccurs. Check the placenta and membranes to make sure they are complete, with no pieces left in the uterus, preventing it from fully contracting.

A potential or uncontrollable hemorrhage, of course, demands *immediate emergency management* from the birth attendant, including medication, bi-manual compression, oxygen, treating shock, and/or transport to the nearest hospital. Use homeopathic remedies in addition to these measures.

There are many homeopathic remedies that are effective in treating a uterine hemorrhage. You need to familiarize yourself with them *prior* to labor, since there is usually not the time during a potential hemorrhage to read through and make a choice. The most important remedy is, of course, the one that is needed for your particular situation. However, I suggest you begin your study with these most commonly used hemorrhagic remedies: *Arnica, Aconite, Caulophyllum, Phosphorus, Hamamelis, Ipecacuanha, Belladonna, Pulsatilla, Sabina, Secale,* and *Sepia*. With time and experience, these remedies and others will become familiar to you.

First Remedy to Consider:

Arnica: Routinely give a high potency dose (200c or whatever you have on hand) during labor and another dose right after birth to prevent hemorrhaging and shock.

Also think of *Arnica* when there has been a very rapid, long or traumatic birth, prolonged or difficult pushing stage, a large baby, shoulder dystocia, or forceps birth. The woman who will benefit from *Arnica* feels bruised and sore all over. The flow is bright-red and may be mixed with clots. Pain may or may not be present. The bed feels too hard and the *Arnica* woman has trouble finding a comfortable position. She does not want to be touched or approached because of the soreness. She wants to be left alone and says there is nothing the matter with her.

Other Remedies to Consider:

Aconite: Overwhelming fear with a gushing or spurting, bright-red, flow. There is anxiety, restlessness, fear of death with a bounding pulse. This woman is sure she will die. The *Aconite* state may originate from a severe fright during the labor or birth.

Arnica: See above under "First Remedy to Consider."

Belladonna: Profuse bleeding, with gushing of *hot*, bright-red blood and clots. The blood coagulates very quickly. The bleeding may stop and start suddenly. She may experience a sensation of pressing outwards or bearing down. Sometimes the blood is dark red and smells offensive. She may have a hot, red, flushed face, red eyes, dilated pupils, and throbbing carotids. She is oversensitive to noise, light, and jarring of the bed. The slightest jarring aggravates her.

Carbo vegetabilis: Dark, oozing hemorrhage from uterine atony. The woman needing *Carbo vegetabilis* is worn out, faints easily, and must have fresh air. She may be unconscious or nearly so. This remedy is known as a "corpse reviver." Her lips, breath, and skin are cold. She is very pale, sometimes blue. She may have cold perspiration, particularly on her forehead. Her pulse is thready and nearly imperceptible. Her breathing is labored and quickened. She is chilly, but must have all the windows open, and wants to be fanned. She can have varicosities of the vulva (see *Hamamelis, Millefolium*). The other main remedy to consider for fainting or shock after hemorrhage is *China* (read about *China* below).

The hemorrhage of *Carbo vegetabilis* tends to be more slow and passive than that of *China*. She tends to be weaker and more run down prior to labor, whereas the collapse of someone needing *China* is more from the hemorrhage itself. The desire for open air and to be fanned is more characteristic of *Carbo vegetabilis*.

Carbo vegetabilis may also have gassy distention of the stomach. She is, unlike *China*, very relieved from burping or passing gas.

Caulophyllum: Think of *Caulophyllum* if the uterus is exhausted (atonic uterus) from a very long or difficult labor and birth. There is generalized weakness, exhaustion, trembling, and nervous exhaustion. There may be a retained placenta because the contractions are too weak to expel it. If she needed it during labor, think of repeating it again here.

China: Hemorrhage from uterine atony (lack of tone). This is accompanied by all the common symptoms of shock: dizziness, ringing in ears, thirst, cold sweat, extreme chilliness, weakness, loss of senses and sight, and fainting. The woman who needs *China* looks pale, perhaps yellow, anemic, with dark blue rings around the eyes. She wants to be fanned. The flow can be intermittent with uterine cramps, colic, and painful distention of the abdomen. (Also consider *Carbo vegetabilis* for fainting or shock after hemorrhage.)

China can have the symptom of gassy distention of the abdomen. She feels bloated, distended, and flatulent, but with no relief from burping or passing gas. With *Carbo vegetabilis*, these same symptoms are there, but she feels much better from burping.

When *China* is the indicated remedy, she tends to be extremely sensitive to external stimulation, such as touch, light, noise, and emotional states. She does not want to be touched, even lightly, but is better from hard pressure. She can be irritable, sensitive, and touchy.

China is also excellent, later in the postpartum period, for persistent weakness or exhaustion after excessive loss of fluids, whether blood, sweat, diarrhea, vomit, or lactation.

Cimicifuga: Labor-like pains cease with the hemorrhage. The *Cimicifuga* type seems fine, then becomes hysterical with the pains. Her physical symptoms alternate back and forth one with another or with her mental or emotional state in an abrupt, jumbled and random fashion. There is passive, profuse, dark, coagulated blood. She often has nervous shivering and trembling.

Cinnamonum: Main remedy for placental abruption (premature separation of the placenta from the uterine wall causing massive bleeding). This is a very serious situation which demands *immediate hospital emergency care*. It is indicated for severe bleeding in a primipara (woman having her first baby) after her first few pains and she is only slightly dilated (probably a placenta abruption).

The bleeding is usually sudden, profuse, and bright-red. It can be continuous and passive. It is indicated for a hemorrhage caused from overlifting, overexertion, a strain, or a misstep.

Crotalus horridus: This remedy is rarely needed, but can save a life if this situation ever arises. It should be in every midwife's bag. Use it for a postpartum hemorrhage so profuse that disseminated intravascular coagulation (DIC) is imminent. The blood loses its ability to clot and tends to be dark and thin. The bleeding may be rapid or continuous oozing. It is as if the blood is dissolving, and the vessels are not able to retain the blood within them. Give the highest potency you have on hand every 2 minutes until the bleeding stops. (Note: DIC is an abnormality in the clotting ability of the blood triggered by excess bleeding and leading to further bleeding.)

Think of *Crotalus horridus* to stop the bleeding of an episiotomy or tear that continuously oozes blood from the slightest provocation. The blood tends to be dark, thin, and without clots. The tissue looks bruised.

Hamamelis: Slow, steady, continuous, dark bleeding (see *Secale*) that oozes out, unclotted, in women with a strong tendency to varicosities, hemorrhoids, and varicose veins. The varicosities and hemorrhoids often feel swollen, sore, and painful. There are no uterine pains with the flow. The woman who *Hamamelis* would benefit usually feels very weak from the slow, steady blood loss. Often, there is a hammering headache, especially about the temples, and she shows no alarm or anxiety about the hemorrhage. Less commonly, the bleeding can be bright-red and come in gushes.

Ipecacuanha: Constant, profuse oozing and gushing of bright-red blood. This woman's face is deathly pale. She feels easily prostrated and faint. She may or may not have nausea with the flow, however, nausea with the flow is a good confirmation for the use of this remedy. There are cutting pains about the umbilicus, darting towards the uterus (opposite direction of *Sepia*). She may breathe heavily, panting and gasping for breath during the hemorrhage. The hemorrhage is worse from motion (see *Sabina, Secale*). She is chilly, shuddering, and has cold sweat especially from the hands and feet. Though usually thirstless, sometimes there is thirst.

Think of *Ipecacuanha* when *Phosphorus* seemed indicated but did not help. It is also an important remedy for hemorrhaging after the removal of the placenta.

Lachesis: The blood tends to be thin, dark and purplish looking. It can even look black and have pieces like charred straw in it. Bleeding is copious and prolonged. An odd symptom is that the *Lachesis* woman feels generally better as soon as the flow begins. The less the flow, the more the pain. She feels pain in her right ovarian region that increases more and more until relieved by a gush of blood.

This woman is very talkative, with a strong need to express herself in order to relieve her inner tension. She frequently jumps from one subject to another. Her nature is emotionally passionate, exploding with anger and jealousy, or sad and gloomy.

While generally very sensitive to touch and pressure, she cannot bear anything touching her throat or having pressure on her abdomen. She is generally worse from lying on her left side, has hot flushes, and likes open air.

Millefolium: Bright-red, profuse hemorrhages that are thin, fluid, sudden, and painless. The flow is continuous. This birthing woman typically experiences no anxiety (for profuse flow of bright-red blood with anxiety and restlessness, think of *Aconite*). She can have painful varicosities during pregnancy that ulcerate and bleed (see *Hamamelis*). It is useful for prolonged obstinate bleeding after a hard labor. The hemorrhage can occur after slight exertion during labor. Dr. J. T. Kent (a prominent American homeopath, 1849-1916) felt that a woman predisposed to hemorrhage should be given a dose of Millefolium before going into labor.

Phosphorus: Copious, bright-red, and thin blood that may or may not have clots, especially true for tall, slender women with a history of easy bleeding (nosebleeds, profuse menstrual bleeding, etc.) and easy bruising. The bleeding may be passive, gushing, continuous, or oozing. The hemorrhage can come on suddenly without obvious cause since the labor was uneventful and the placenta delivered complete.

The *Phosphorus* woman has an unquenchable thirst

for ice cold water. She is usually chilly (not always) and sensitive to cold.

The mental-emotional state does not have to be there, but is an excellent confirmation for the use of this remedy. This type of woman tends to be very sensitive, empathic, affectionate, and desires company. She is also anxious and fearful, especially when alone or in the dark, but is easily reassured. She often feels "spacey." She loves massage, touch, and lots of affection. The characteristic *Phosphorus* woman is tall, thin, and delicate, with long fingers.

If *Phosphorus* seems indicated but does not act, try *Ipecacuanha*.

Pulsatilla: For a postpartum hemorrhage often secondary to retained placenta or blood clots. The symptoms change in character; profuse, intermittent blood which can be dark, clotted, thick, or thin, and watery. The hemorrhage alternates with labor-pains.

Think of *Pulsatilla* for the woman who has a strong need for affection, attention, approval, and reassurance from others. Her emotions are on the surface. She is easily moved to tears and feels much better from crying. She tends to be soft, sweet, affectionate, and sympathetic. She wants plenty of fresh air and probably will have the windows wide open.

Read more about *Pulsatilla* in the chapter "Prolonged, Difficult, or Dysfunctional Labor."

Sabina: Active, gushing, bright-red, thin flow, mixed with clots, usually accompanied by a lot of cramping or pain. The clots can be large and are typically dark colored. Less often the blood may be dark. The pains can be extreme. They begin in the low back or sacrum and extend to the pubis. This woman often complains of pains when trying to expel clots. The slightest motion increases the flow (see *Ipecacuanha, Secale*), but may be paradoxically better from walking. The bleeding starts when she takes a deep breath. There may be a retained placenta.

She is intolerant of warm air and a warm room, and desires cool open air (see *Pulsatilla, Secale*). Her face flushes and is florid. She is aggravated by music which makes her nervous.

The bleeding is similar to *Belladonna, Ipecacuanha,* and *Phosphorus*.

Secale: For passive, continuous trickling bleeding (see *Hamamelis*) that can add up to a substantial blood loss if the bleeding is not stopped. The uterus has no tone and contracts only temporarily with massage. The blood is often dark, liquid, unclotted, and may be offensive. The flow increases with the slightest motion (see *Ipecacuanha, Sabina*). There may be no pain or bearing down pains. She also may have hourglass contractions, tetanic contractions, and violent, irregular contractions that prevent the placenta from descending. The woman who *Secale* will benefit feels burning hot and cannot tolerate covers, though her skin may be cold to touch. She feels better from open air, being fanned, cold, and from uncovering.

She may experience tingling all over her skin with the hemorrhage and want to be rubbed. A strange symptom of the *Secale* woman is being very bothered if her fingers touch each other, forcing her to hold her fingers spread apart.

Secale is especially indicated for the woman who has had a number of children close together (see *Sepia*).

She is often thin and feels weak and exhausted. Her uterus has no tone and contracts only temporarily with massage. Excruciating afterpains may be experienced, especially when the baby nurses. Midwife and homeopath, Pat Kramer, refers to *Secale* as the "homeopathic methergine." (Methergine is a drug used in obstetrics to stimulate a sustained, tetanic contraction of the uterus.)

Sepia: For hemorrhaging when there is a strong bearing down sensation. She feels as if her uterus is going to fall out of her vagina and may cross her legs to keep this from happening. There is a sense of weight in her anus like a heavy ball. She has fine darting pains in her cervix from below upward and feels better from drawing up her legs.

The *Sepia* woman is chilly and sensitive to the cold, with flushes of heat. She likes being covered up warmly (the opposite of *Secale*). There often are yellow or brown spots on her face (chloasma) or a yellow saddle across her nose.

Emotionally she feels indifferent and detached from her family and the new baby because she is tired and worn out. She is not attentive to her newborn, even when the baby cries. She feels very tired. Her impulse is to want to be left alone and not be bothered by demands or responsibilities. However, the *Sepia* woman typically dreads being completely alone. In extreme cases, she feels angry and hateful towards the newborn with a desire to hurt the child. These feelings may scare and horrify her. This state reminds us of a woman who has a number of children and then is unexpectedly pregnant again. The pregnancy is not wanted. The mental-emotional state does not have to be there to prescribe *Sepia*, but is a good confirmation for the choice of this remedy.

Sepia is an excellent remedy for the prevention and treatment of actual uterine prolapse. It is also excellent for postpartum depression when she feels detached from, or even hates, her baby and husband/partner.

Trillium: Active or passive hemorrhage from lack of uterine tone in an obese, flabby woman. This woman feels like her hips and back are falling to pieces (breaking). She feels very faint and dizzy. There is a gush of bright blood on the least movement. The discharge is profuse, thick, and dark clotted. There are bearing down sensations, especially if she stands or walks. Tightly bandaging her pelvis helps her to feel better. She has a history of hemorrhaging after every birth.

Ustilago: Passive, slow, and persistent hemorrhage of dark blood with small black clots, from lack of uterine tone (atonic uterus). The blood is part fluid and part clots. It is semifluid, but not watery. Oozing of dark clotted blood can form long black strings. The bleeding can be of bright-red clots accompanied by a bearing down sensation. Her uterus feels as though it is drawn up into a knot. Her cervix is spongy and bleeds easily. Her blood may smell very offensive (putrid). A vaginal exam brings on oozing of blood with small black clots. She tends to weep frequently and feel depressed.

Repertory for Postpartum Hemorrhage

(An explanation of repertory structure and remedy grading can be found in the beginning of the "Repertory For Prolonged, Difficult, or Dysfunctional Labor," page 61. See the remedy index at the back of the book for remedy abbreviations.)

POSTPARTUM HEMORRHAGE: *Arn., Acon., Bell., Carb-v., Caul., Chin., Cimic., Cinnm., Crot-h., Ham., Ip., Lach., Mill., Phos., Puls., Sabin., Sec., Sep., Tril., Ust.*
Canth., Gels., Goss., Ign., Kali-c., Plat. are written about in other chapters. Check the "Remedy Index" in back of the book.

FAINTING: See "Shock/Fainting" below.

MENTAL AND EMOTIONAL SYMPTOMS: See the repertory for "Prolonged, Difficult, or Dysfunctional Labor" for a more complete mental and emotional symptoms listing. The following two symptoms are for remedies not covered in that chapter and repertory.
Talkative (loquacious) and passionate, must talk to relieve her inner tension: Lach.
Weeps frequently and is depressed: Ust.

POSTPARTUM HEMORRHAGE (metrorrhagia):
Abruption, placental (premature separation of the placenta from the uterine wall causing massive bleeding): Cinnm.
Active: See "Gushing" and "Profuse" below.
After:
Difficult labor, in tall and slender women: Phos.

After (continued):

    Precipitous birth (very fast): Arn., Caul.

    Traumatic birth, with soreness and
        bruising: Arn.

Air, desire for open: Acon., **Puls.**, <u>Sabin.</u>, <u>Sec.</u>

Atonic uterus, with (uterine inertia): Carb-v.,
    Caul., Chin., Puls., Sabin., Sec., Sep., Tril.,
    <u>Ust.</u>

    Fall out, feels as if everything is going to,
        out of her uterus and vagina: Sep.

    Obese, flabby women, in, with history of
        hemorrhaging after every birth: Tril.

    Pain, extreme, from sacrum to pubis,
        complains of, when expelling clots:
        Sabin.

    Weak, run down, prior to labor, depleted to
        the point of collapse: Carb-v.

    Weakness, exhaustion, and trembling, with:
        Caul.

    Women who have had many children close
        together: Sec., Sep.

        Air, desire for open: Sec.

        Chilly and desires to be covered: Sep.

        Hot and cannot tolerate being covered:
        Sec.

Better, feels, as soon as the flow begins: Lach.

Bleeding and bruising, history of easy: Phos.

Bright-red: Acon., Arn., Bell., Cinnm., <u>Ip.</u>, Mill.,
    Phos., Sabin., <u>Ust.</u>

    Abruption, placenta, from: Cinnm.

    Die, sure she is going to: Acon.

    Fluid and painless: Mill.

Ceasing for a few moments, then renews with
    redoubled force: Puls.

Ceasing suddenly and suddenly returns: Bell.

Changeable symptoms in color and flow: Puls.

Clotted: Phos., <u>Sabin.</u>, <u>Tril.</u>
Coagulates quickly, sudden, profuse, and hot:
    Bell.
Constant: <u>Ip.</u>, <u>Ust.</u>, Sec.
Copious: See "Profuse" below.
Dark: Bell., Carb-v., Caul., Chin., Cimic.,
    Crot-h., <u>Gels.</u>, Ham., <u>Ip.</u>, Lach., <u>Sabin.</u>, Sec.,
    Tril., <u>Ust.</u>
    Better, feels, as soon as the flow begins:
        Lach.
    Fluid: Sec.
    Passive, slow bleeding with small black
        clots, that may form long black strings:
        Ust.
    Purplish or black looking, maybe with
        pieces like charred straw in it: Lach.
    Varicosities (varicose veins), with a strong
        tendency to, which feel swollen and
        painful: Ham.
Easy and sudden bleeding of bright-red blood
    without any cause: Phos.
    When Phos. does not act: Ip.
Fall out, feels as if everything is going to, out of
    her uterus and vagina: Sep.
First remedy to consider: Arn.
Gushing: Acon., <u>Bell.</u>, **Ip.**, **Phos.**, <u>Puls.</u>, **Sabin.**,
    <u>Sec.</u>, Tril. <u>Ust.</u> (See "Profuse" below.)
    Bleeding and bruising, history of easy:
        Phos.
    Changeable symptoms in color and flow:
        Puls.
    Cutting pain about the umbilicus, with: Ip.
    Die, sure she is going to: Acon.
    Fear, with overwhelming: Acon.
    Hot blood: Bell., Ip.
        Face, hot and flushed: Bell.
        Face, pale: Ip.

Gushing, hot blood (continued):
    Pain and cramping, with a lot of, from low
        back or sacrum extending to the pubis:
        Sabin.
    Profuse: Ham., **Ip.**
Hot: Bell., Ip.
    Face, hot and flushed: Bell
    Face, pale: Ip.
    Profuse, in gushes: Bell.
Intermittent flow: <u>Bell.</u>, <u>Cham.</u>, Chin., <u>Ip.</u>,
    Nux-v., **Phos.**, <u>Puls.</u>, <u>Sabin.</u>, Sec., Ust.
    Alternating with labor pains: Puls.
    Ceases for a few moments, then renews
        with redoubled force: Puls.
    Pouring out freely, then ceasing for a short
        time: Phos.
    Uterine cramps, with, colic and painful
        distention of abdomen: Chin.
Jar, aggravated from least: Bell., Ham.
Motion, slightest, aggravates: Ip., Cinnm.,
    Sabin., Sec., Tril.
    Abruption, placenta or from overlifting:
        Cinnm.
    Body temperature:
        Chilly and pale: Ip.
        Hot: Sabin., Sec.
    Obese, flabby women, in, with history of
        hemorrhaging after every birth: Tril.
    Walking, flow better from: Sabin.
Nausea, with: Ip.
Overlifting, overexertion, a strain, or a misstep,
    from: Cinnm.
Pain, girdle-like, from sacrum to pubis,
    complains of, when expelling clots: Sabin.
Pain, labor, cease with the hemorrhage: Cimic.,
    Puls.

Passive: Carb-v., Caul., Chin., Cimic., Ham., Phos., Sec., Tril., Ust.

Slow bleeding of dark blood with small black clots that may form long black strings: Ust.

Trickle, constant, in women who have had many children close together: Sec.

Varicosities (varicose veins), with a strong tendency to, which feel swollen and painful: Ham.

Placenta, from retained: <u>Bell.</u>, <u>Canth.</u>, <u>Carb-v.</u>, Caul., Goss., <u>Ip.</u>, <u>Kali-c.</u>, <u>Puls.</u>, <u>Sabin.</u>, Sec., Sep., Ust. (See "Repertory for Retained Placenta" in that chapter.)

Profuse, speedily coagulating blood: Bell.

Prevents hemorrhage: <u>Arn.</u>

Profuse: Arn., Acon., <u>Bell.</u>, <u>Caul.</u>, <u>Chin.</u>, Cimic., <u>Cinnm.</u>, Crot-h., <u>Ham.</u>, **Ip.**, Mill., Lach., **Phos.**, <u>Plat.</u>, Puls., <u>Sabin.</u>, <u>Sec.</u>, Tril., Ust. (See "Gushing" above.)

Abruption, placenta, from: Cinnm.

Better, feels, as soon as the flow begins: Lach.

Bleeding and bruising, history of easy: Phos.

Changeable symptoms in color and flow: Puls.

Coagulates quickly, sudden, profuse, and hot: Bell.

Continuous: Arn., Ham., **Ip.**, Mill., Phos., Sec., Ust.

DIC (disseminated intravascular coagulation) is imminent: Crot-h.

Die, sure she is going to: Acon.

Easy and sudden bleeding of bright-red blood without any cause: Phos.

When Phos. does not act: Ip.

Faintness and collapse, with symptoms of: Ip.

Profuse (continued):
  Haughty with delusion of superiority: <u>Plat.</u>
  Pain and cramping, with a lot of, from low
      back or sacrum extending to the pubis:
      Sabin.
  Pouring out freely, then ceasing for a short
      time: Phos.
  Purplish or black looking, maybe with
      pieces like charred straw in it: Lach.
  Shock, with symptoms of: Chin.
  Traumatic birth, after, with soreness and
      bruising: Arn.
  Unclotted and so profuse that DIC
      (disseminated intravascular
      coagulation) is imminent: Crot-h.
Protracted (long lasting): Arn., Sec.
  Uterine atony, from: Sec.
Purplish or black looking, maybe with pieces
    like charred straw in it: Lach.
Shock: See "Shock/Fainting" below.
Smells offensive (putrid): <u>Ust.</u>
Strings, long black: Ust.
Sudden, profuse, hot, and coagulates quickly:
    Bell.
Thirst, unquenchable, for ice cold water, with:
    Phos.
Traumatic birth, after, with soreness and
    bruising: Arn.
Varicosities (varicose veins), with a strong
    tendency to, which feel swollen and
    painful: Ham.

SHOCK/FAINTING:
  Faint, feels: Carbo-v., Chin., Ip., Tril.
    Obese, flabby women with history of
        hemorrhaging after every birth: Tril.

Faint, feels (continued):
  Shock, and: Carbo-v., Chin. (See "Shock"
    below.)
Gas in stomach, with: Carb-v., Chin.
  Burping does not relieve: Chin.
  Burping relieves: Carb-v.
Shock, two main remedies for: Carb-v., Chin.
  Air, open, desire for: <u>Carbo-v.</u>, Chin.
    And to be fanned: <u>Carbo-v.</u>, Chin.
  Sensitivity, extreme, to stimulation: Chin.
  Weak, run down, prior to labor: Carb-v.

CHAPTER 12

Retained Placenta

The placenta usually detaches from the uterine wall with the first few contractions following the birth of the baby. There can be a normal delay of 10 to 30 minutes. When the placenta separates from the uterine wall you will see a separation gush of blood and a lengthening of the cord as the placenta descends. As the birth attendant, you will be monitoring the bleeding to make sure it is not excessive. You should encourage the new mother to push when her placenta is fully detached and she is having a contraction. Squatting can help by adding the force of gravity.

The best approach to promote the delivery of the placenta is putting the newborn to the breast to nurse immediately following birth. Some babies latch on right away and need no assistance, while most need some help and encouragement. Just having the baby's mouth on her nipple will help the new mother to produce more oxytocin, causing her uterus to contract more strongly, thus expelling the placenta. She or her partner can also stimulate her nipples if the baby is not yet interested in sucking.

The birth attendant needs to be patient and gentle in delivering the placenta, while closely monitoring the bleeding. *Never yank on the cord or massage the uterus prior to the placenta delivering.* This can cause massive hemorrhaging.

Remedies useful for hemorrhaging are also useful for expelling a retained placenta, since both tend to occur simultaneously. Look at the remedies mentioned in the chapter "Postpartum Hemorrhage."

Remedies to Consider:

Belladonna: Retained placenta with profuse flow of hot blood which coagulates quickly. The slightest jar causes the *Belladonna* woman to suffer. Her face is red and hot. Her skin in general, as well as her vagina, is dry and hot. She is often greatly distressed and moans.

Cantharis: Retained placenta or membranes with a constant desire to urinate. However, the woman who *Cantharis* would benefit typically is only able to pass a few drops of urine or none at all, and it is painful to do so. Burning or cutting pains are felt in the bladder, kidney, pelvis, vagina or back. The cervix often is swollen from labor.

Caulophyllum: When labor and birth have been long and exhausting and there is not enough energy left to push the placenta out. The uterus is hypotonic (does not stay contracted). There is generalized weakness, exhaustion, trembling, and nervous exhaustion. If she needed it during labor, think of repeating it again here.

Cimicifuga: Retained placenta with dysfunctional uterine contractions, severe tearing pains, or no uterine activity, rheumatic pains in the back and limbs, and irrational fears, anxiety, and nervous agitation.

Typically, this woman experiences nervous shivering and trembling. The physical symptoms alternate back and forth with one another or with mental or emotional states in an abrupt, jumbled, and random fashion. Labor-like pains cease with the hemorrhage. She seems fine, then becomes hysterical with the pains.

Gossypium: This is the main remedy for placenta accreta, where the placenta is firmly attached to the walls of the uterus and will not detach. Also think of it for a retained placenta after a premature delivery when the placenta will not detach no matter what is done. No amount of force seems sufficient to dislodge it.

Pulsatilla: A commonly used remedy for retained placenta. Think of *Pulsatilla* for the woman who has a strong need for affection, attention, approval, and reassurance from others. Her emotions are on the surface. She is easily moved to tears and feels much better from crying. She tends to be soft, sweet, affectionate, and sympathetic. She wants plenty of fresh air and will have the windows wide open.

Pulsatilla is also the first remedy to use for retained placenta when there are no guiding symptoms that lead to the choice of another remedy. *Sepia* is the second.

Read more about *Pulsatilla* in the chapter "Prolonged, Difficult, or Dysfunctional Labor."

Sabina: Retained placenta with active, bright-red bleeding, partly fluid, partly clotted, worsening with every motion, and with severe afterpains. There is pain from the sacrum to the pubis. She complains of girdle-like pains from the sacrum around to the pubis when trying to expel clots. There is a discharge of fluid blood and clots in equal parts, with each contraction. The hemorrhage is often complicated by a retained placenta.

The *Sabina* woman is aggravated by music, which makes her nervous. She is also intolerant of warm air and a warm room, and desires cool open air (see *Pulsatilla*, *Secale*).

Secale: Retained placenta with a constant, strong sensation of bearing down (see *Sepia*). The hemorrhage is continuous and passive, often with dark, thin, unclotted blood. The flow increases with the slightest motion (see *Sabina*). The *Secale* type has contractions which are weak or absent because the uterus is weak and exhausted. Her uterus has no tone. She may also have hourglass contractions, tetanic contractions, and violent, irregular contractions that prevent the placenta from descending. Similar to *Sepia*, *Secale* is often needed in thin, weak women who have had a lot of children.

Secale, unlike *Sepia*, is very hot and cannot tolerate covers, though her skin may be cold to touch. She feels better from open air, being fanned, cold, and from uncovering.

Sepia: Her pelvis feels congested with a sensation of heaviness. There is a strong bearing down sensation, as if her uterus is going to fall out of her vagina. She may cross her legs to keep this from happening. Also, she may have little, sharp, shooting pains in the cervix, sometimes with burning. Hourglass contractions prevent the placenta from descending. She is chilly, has cold hands and feet, is sensitive to the cold, but has flushes of heat. She likes to be covered warmly (opposite of *Secale*).

Sepia is the second remedy to use for retained placenta when there are no guiding symptoms that lead to the choice of another remedy. *Pulsatilla* is the first.

See the chapter "Prolonged, Difficult, or Dysfunctional Labor" for the mental-emotional state of *Sepia*.

Repertory for Retained Placenta

(An explanation of repertory structure and remedy grading can be found in the beginning of the "Repertory For Prolonged, Difficult, or Dysfunctional Labor," page 61. See the remedy index at the back of the book for remedy abbreviations.)

RETAINED PLACENTA: *Bell., Canth., Caul., Cimic., Goss., Puls., Sabin., Sec., Sep.*
Arn., Ars., Chin., Cinnm., Gels., Ip., Plat. are written about in other chapters. Check the "Remedy Index" in back of the book.
Abruption, placental (premature separation of the placenta from the uterine wall causing massive bleeding): Cinnm.
Accreta, placenta: Goss.
Adherent: Goss., Puls.
Firmly, force will hardly dislodge it: Goss.
Air, desire for open: **Puls.**, Sabin., Sec.
Bearing down, with constant strong: Sec., Sep.
Contractions of uterus:
Absent: Caul., Cimic., Puls.
Deficient (inadequate): Ip., Puls., Sec.
Imperfect or else very prolonged: Sec.
Control, need to have everything in, with nervous restlessness and anxiety: Ars.
Exhaustion, from a long and exhausting labor and birth: Arn., Caul.
Feverishness, with: Bell., Canth.
Genitalia, external, very sensitive, cannot tolerate anything touching her genitalia: Plat.
Hemorrhage, with uterine: Bell., Caul., Chin., Ip., Plat., Puls., Sabin., Sec. (See "Repertory for Postpartum Hemorrhage" in that chapter.)

Hysterical as soon as the contractions start, fine in
    between: Cimic.
Jar, slight, causes suffering: Bell.
Nausea, with: Ip.
Pain:
    Cutting pain, in lower abdomen, running
        upward, or upward and backward: Gels.
    Distressing, tearing pain in uterine region, with
        no uterine action: Cimic.
    Intense, very: Sabin.
    Sharp pinching pains, about the umbilicus,
        running to the uterus: Ip.
    Sharp, shooting pains in cervix, at times with
        burning: Sep.
Profuse flow:
    Of bright-red hot blood which coagulates
        quickly: Bell.
    Of bright-red or dark fluid blood and clots in
        equal parts, with girdle-like pains from
        sacrum around to pubis, when trying to
        expel clots: Sabin.
Symptoms, no guiding, that lead to the choice of
    another remedy:
    First remedy to use: Puls.
    Second remedy to use: Sep.
Urination, with painful: Canth.
Uterine atony (lack of tone), from: Arn., Caul.,
    <u>Puls.</u>, Sec., Sep.
    Exhaustion, from a long and exhausting labor
        and birth: Arn., Caul.
    Want of expulsive power: Caul., <u>Puls.</u>
    Women who have had a number of children
        close together: Sec., Sep.
        Air, desire for open: Sec.
        Chilly and desires to be covered: Sep.
        Hot and cannot tolerate being covered: Sec.

Vagina, with heat and dryness of: Bell.
Vomiting, with: Canth., Ip.
Want of expulsive power: See "Uterine atony, from" above.
Warmth, distressed by: Sec.
Weeping, because the labor is not completed: <u>Puls.</u>

CHAPTER 13

Postpartum Infections

A postpartum infection is an unlikely occurrence if the birthing woman is healthy and basic hygiene is adhered to during the labor and birth. This is even more true for a homebirth since she has already developed antibodies to most of the germs in her home environment. She has not been exposed to the numerous pathogenic germs (germs that produce disease) present in the hospital.

Symptoms of a uterine infection include a temperature over 100.4° F., foul discharge, elevated pulse, pelvic or abdominal tenderness or pain, subinvolution of the uterus, aching, and chills. (Note: Subinvolution is when the uterus fails to reduce to normal size following childbirth.)

The main cause of an elevated temperature in the first 24 hours following birth is dehydration. This is especially true if there has been a significant blood loss. Be sure the new mother drinks lots of fluids during labor and postpartum. I suggest that she drink a tall glass of fluid every time she nurses the newborn, which is about every 2 hours.

The new mom is at risk of a postpartum infection if she has had:

- prolonged labor, especially with ruptured membranes

- prolonged rupture of the membranes (over 24 hours)

- repeated vaginal exams, especially with ruptured membranes

- manual removal of the placenta

- manual exploration of the uterus

- delayed delivery of the placenta

- retained placental parts or membranes

- extensive tissue trauma

- hemorrhage, or

- surgical delivery, such as a cesarean section.

Another cause of postpartum infection is over-activity and exhaustion in the first postpartum days. Be sure the new mom is on bedrest and otherwise taking it easy in order to let her body heal and make all the adjustments that occur postpartum. This is a special time for her to just be with her precious newborn.

The temperature of the postpartum woman can also elevate when her milk is about to come in and for a couple of days following. Again, encourage her to drink lots of fluids and monitor for the other symptoms of postpartum infection.

The new mother must be made aware that if a postpartum infection is suspected, she should notify her midwife immediately. The following remedy can be used while she is being evaluated and monitored:

Pyrogenium: *Pyrogenium* is almost a specific for post-partum infections. If a postpartum infection seems imminent (fever, chills, or a foul smelling flow), give a dose of *Pyrogenium* immediately. It will usually abort the infection before further symptoms develop.

Use a 200c dose once and then only as needed if the symptoms return. If you are using a 30c potency, give a dose every 15 minutes for an hour, every hour for 3 hours, then 3 times a day for a few days as needed. Stop when the symptoms are gone. You should see the temperature going down and an overall improvement of symptoms within a few hours or less of taking the correct remedy.

In a more advanced postpartum infection, *Pyrogenium* symptoms include aching and soreness with fever, highly offensive discharge and lochia (postpartum blood flow), and a disparity between the pulse rate and the temperature. A characteristic symptom indicating the need for *Pyrogenium* is when the pulse rate is high while there is only a moderate fever, or the pulse rate is low with a high fever.

CHAPTER 14

Injuries to the Coccyx and Spine

During labor, the coccyx (tailbone) is sometimes bruised and displaced. An injury to the coccyx or spine can cause severe, long lasting pain. Causes of nerve damage include a forceps delivery, epidural, or other injection. (Note: An epidural is the injection of epidural anesthesia into the space between the wall of the vertebral canal and the membranes—three in all—that cover the spinal cord and contain the spinal fluid. An epidural can be effective for control of labor pain by numbing the lower part of the body, but it is not without risks to mother and baby.) The dangers of epidural anesthesia are many, and it is the right of every pregnant woman to be advised of these prior to labor in order to make an informed decision. Epidural anesthesia significantly reduces the ability of the uterus to contract effectively, resulting in a slower rate of cervical dilation and a longer second stage. This leads to the increased use of oxytocin, forceps, cesarean delivery, and the risks inherent in these procedures.

Another common complication of epidurals is when one or more of the membranes and its associated nerves is accidentally punctured during insertion of the needle. This often results in numbness, motor weakness, pain, headaches, and other symptoms.

Other potential risks include nausea, vomiting, a serious drop in maternal blood pressure, respiratory arrest, cardiac arrest, as well as numerous fetal and newborn complications.

Epidural anesthesia for normal labor increases the necessity of further medical intervention. The International Childbirth Education Association (ICEA) holds the position that, as with all obstetrical tests, technologies, and procedures, epidural anesthesia should not be routinely recommended for laboring women, but instead reserved for situations where the perceived benefits of its use outweigh the known and perceived risks.

If the new mother's coccyx feels sore, it may have gotten pushed back during the birth of the baby's head and be out of place. The following exercise can soothe and alleviate the soreness:

Have the new mom lie on her stomach (a wonderful new experience now that the baby is born!). Her partner or a friend, while straddling her legs, should place his/her hand along the postpartum woman's spine with the heel of his/her palm cupped on her coccyx and his/her fingers on the spine in the direction of her head. The partner's other hand should be on top of the first hand. Have him/her place continuous *gentle* pressure downwards against the mother's coccyx (towards the floor) with the heel of his/her palm (using both hands) for as long as it is soothing. This can be repeated twice a day for a few days, or as often as desired. The new mom may also want to see a chiropractor for a professional adjustment.

Remedies to Consider:

Arnica: When the new mother feels sore and bruised in one area of her body or all over. She does not want to be touched or approached because she is so sore. She is restless in bed, saying it is too hard, and cannot find a comfortable position.

Use a 30c potency three times a day for a few days or until the soreness is alleviated.

Hypericum: This is the main remedy for traumatic injuries to parts that are rich in nerves, such as the coccyx and spine. The pains are intense and sensitive to touch. They shoot from the injury along the course of wounded nerves, towards the trunk, up the spine, or down the legs. Use a 30c potency every 15 minutes for an hour, every hour for 3 hours, then 3 times a day for several days, or as needed for pain. A dose can be given every few minutes, as needed, if the pain is excruciating. *Hypericum* can resolve the pain quickly even if given years after the original injury.

Ledum: *Ledum* is an important remedy for puncture wounds. Think of it for pain and complications after an epidural (read the footnote on epidural anesthesia in the beginning of this chapter) or lumbar puncture. *Ledum* is particularly indicated when the injured area feels cold to the touch, or is greatly ameliorated by cold application and aggravated by heat.

Use 30c, 200c, or 1M as needed for pain. A 30c potency can be given as instructed for *Hypericum*, above. With a 200c or 1M potency, a healing response should be seen soon after a single dose. It may need to be repeated a few times again if the symptoms return.

Ledum follows *Arnica* well for traumatic injuries with bruising and soreness when *Arnica* has done all that it can. A 30c potency is sufficient for this purpose.

CHAPTER 15

Preventing and Healing a Perineal Tear or Episiotomy

In my experience, I have found that episiotomies are surgical interventions usually unnecessary in the natural birth process. They are painful, traumatizing, difficult to control, cause needless bleeding, and take a long time to heal. Episiotomies are necessary only in about 1% of births—for emergencies only. In these cases, they are a lifesaving measure.

There are effective methods for increasing the health and elasticity of the pregnant woman's perineal tissues prior to the birth, thus increasing the possibility of birthing the baby without an episiotomy or tear. These include good nutrition (the first line of defense for healthy, stretchy tissue, and improved ability to heal), daily pelvic floor exercise throughout pregnancy, and perineal massage during the last month of pregnancy. (Note: See appendices for instructions on pelvic floor/Kegel exercise and perineal massage.) Both pelvic floor exercise and perineal massage increase the blood flow, health, and elasticity of this area. Both help the expectant mother to identify the muscles of the pelvic floor and to learn to relax them in response to pressure. This is of obvious benefit as the baby is being born. Perineal massage stretches the perineal tissues making more room for the baby to be born. Massaging oil into the perineum softens the tissue, again reducing resistance.

Supporting the perineal tissues during the birth in order to prevent or minimize tearing is an art which has been handed down from midwife to midwife. It is not taught in medical school. Be sure the birth attendant has the necessary knowledge and experience. Warm cloths and oil are used to keep the perineum relaxed and well lubricated. The same bottle of oil used for perineal massage can be used here. Some women choose to labor and give birth (or just labor) in a warm tub of water. These water births greatly assist with relaxation and minimize tearing. Good communication and trust between the pregnant woman and her birth attendant is an absolute necessity to help birth the baby slowly, allowing the tissues to stretch as needed.

Often women do get what are called "skid marks," small superficial splits in the tissue of the labia. These can be very tender as it is the superficial tissues that contain the most nerves. Other times, even with the best of care and intention, tears occur. To reiterate, in emergencies, where the life of the baby is in danger, an episiotomy becomes a lifesaving measure. The following remedies will help greatly in the healing of these wounds.

Remedies to Consider:

Arnica: *Arnica* will promote healing, control bleeding, prevent and reduce swelling, soreness, bruising, and prevent infections after a perineal tear or episiotomy.
It is particularly indicated if the new mother's

bottom feels sore and bruised. She does not want to be touched there. Her chair and bed feel too hard. It is uncomfortable for her to sit up or have anything touching her bottom. She cannot find a comfortable position.

Use a 30c three times a day for up to a week or 200c once a day for up to a few days until the swelling and soreness are gone.

If swelling is extreme, or just to experience a soothing pack, apply ice packs to the perineum along with taking *Arnica*. Many mothers find ice packs extremely refreshing after giving birth. A quick ice pack can be made by filling a sterile glove with crushed ice and tying off the end. Put a sterile gauze pad on the side that will be next to the perineum and give it a squirt of clean calendula or olive oil (or whatever oil was used for the birth). This prevents the pack from sticking to the skin.

Ice packs should not be applied for longer than 24 hours, except in the event of a hematoma which is enlarging. After 24 hours, some women who have had stitches enjoy exposing the stitches to a high wattage light bulb for a few minutes. Be careful the woman does not sit too close to the bulb or expose the area for too long as this can burn the perineum! Use extreme care if an infrared heat lamp is used.

Calendula: *Calendula* is excellent used as an antiseptic and to help the layers of torn skin 'knit' back together. It will soothe pain, stop bleeding, promote healing, prevent scarring, and prevent infection.

Use it routinely as a lotion when there has been any tearing. You may use *Calendula* topically even when another indicated homeopathic remedy, orally in potency, is taken.

Make a lotion by adding either 1/2 teaspoon (2 - 3 dropperfuls) of *Calendula tincture* or 2 teaspoons of *Calendula succus* or *Calendula nonalcoholic* to 8 ounces of warm water. Lotions do not keep, so make some daily as needed. It is useful to have a peribottle (an 8 ounce squirt bottle) to easily apply the lotion by squirting it on. Use this lotion to carefully clean the wound. *Calendula* promotes rapid healing from the outside in, so it can seal dirt into the body, if the wound is not carefully cleaned. (Note: All forms of *Calendula* are effective in promoting the healing of wounds. *Calendula tincture* is prepared in alcohol and therefore, it must be greatly diluted to not sting or burn delicate or raw tissue. *Calendula nonalcoholic* is prepared with glycerine. *Calendula succus* is the juice of the plant with a minimal amount of alcohol added.)

Calendula lotion will not cause the irritation common to conventional antiseptics. Do not, however, use the tincture undiluted on an open wound, as the alcohol base will burn the raw tissue.

To prevent infections, promote healing, and soothe injured tissues, instruct the new mother to spray the perineal area with the warm *Calendula* lotion each time after going to the bathroom and gently pat (don't rub) dry. She may prefer to spray the warm lotion *while* she is urinating, as the warmth soothes the pain. *Calendula* can also be added to a sitz bath.

A dressing saturated with *Calendula* lotion stops bleeding when applied to cervical or vaginal tears. Be sure to use a sterile dressing such as a cotton gauze pad.

Along with using the lotion, give *Calendula* orally (when another remedy is not needed) in a 30c potency three times a day for a few days to a week, to hasten the healing of injured tissue, and to prevent infection. It is excellent for tears, whether stitched or not, that are having a hard time healing. The pain may be excessive in proportion to the injury. (Also read *Staphysagria* below for second to fourth degree tears.)

Calendula cream is excellent for many types of skin problems including sore or cracked nipples (apply it after nursing) and diaper rash. It is quickly absorbed by the skin and washes off easily.

Crotalus horridus: Think of *Crotalus horridus* to stop the bleeding of an episiotomy or tear that continuously oozes blood from the slightest provocation. The blood tends to be dark, thin, and without clots. The tissue looks bruised.

Read more about *Crotalus horridus* in the chapter, "Postpartum Hemorrhage."

Hypericum: This is the main remedy for injuries to parts that are rich in nerves, so it is useful for pain after a perineal tear (for an episiotomy, use *Staphysagria* instead). *Hypericum* is called for when the pains are intense and shoot along the course of wounded nerves. It will alleviate the pain, promote healing, and prevent infection. Also excellent for injuries to the coccyx or spine with such shooting pains. Other causes may be trauma from childbirth, forceps delivery, epidural, or other injections.

Give *Arnica* first for swelling and bruising, then follow with *Hypericum*, if indicated for pain. If the pain is extreme, however, begin immediately with *Hypericum*. Give a 30c potency every 15 minutes for an hour, every hour for 3 hours, then 3 times a day for several days, or as needed for pain. *Hypericum* can be given every few minutes, for a few doses, if the pain is excruciating.

Staphysagria: This remedy is specific for clean surgical wounds such as episiotomies. It helps these wounds to heal rapidly, while minimizing pain, and preventing infections. Use it instead of *Hypericum* as described above.

Also think of it for a second to fourth degree tear that is painful and not healing, especially if the woman feels she has been violated, humiliated, or assaulted during her labor and birth. She feels emotionally sensitive and her physical wound is sensitive also. The anger will often be suppressed. She may feel guilt or shame instead of angry. She feels disappointed or is resentful. There may be a previous history of incest or sexual abuse. (Note: A first degree tear/laceration involves the perineal skin just below or the vaginal mucosa just inside the opening of the vagina. A second degree tear extends to include the perineal muscles— which ones depend on the depth of the tear. A third degree tear extends into the anal sphincter muscle. A fourth degree tear goes through the anal sphincter and into the anterior rectal wall.)

CHAPTER 16

Healing From a Difficult Delivery or Cesarean Section

Problems can occur in the birth process even when everyone involved has done their best to prevent them. When a cesarean section or other emergency intervention is necessary, it is a lifesaving procedure. Modern medical technology is important and appropriate when these emergencies occur.

It is unfortunate, however, that in the United States, as well as in many other parts of the world, far too many cesareans are done unnecessarily. Many, if not most, of the cesareans performed could be prevented. The irony is that often cesareans become necessary *as a result of* obstetrical interventions, invasive procedures, and negative attitudes about women, pregnancy, and birth that undermine a woman's natural ability to give birth. Women are misled into thinking that "modern medicine" is needed to save a baby's life when, in fact, it is "modern medicine," in these situations, that interferes with Nature's plan.

There are a number of actions that every pregnant woman can take to make sure her birth will be as safe, gentle, and non-invasive as possible. She should:

- Take responsibility for her own pregnancy and birth. She must not expect her midwife or doctor to make her decisions for her.

- Write out a formal birth plan for herself and her baby, and discuss it with her midwife or doctor. The midwife or doctor should sign the birth plan showing agreement to follow it.

- Educate herself thoroughly about cesarean prevention. (I strongly recommend that she read *Silent Knife: Cesarean Prevention & Vaginal Birth After Cesarean*, by Nancy Wainer Cohen and Lois J. Estner. It is an excellent book on cesarean prevention and will cover much more than I am able to here.)

- Take childbirth education classes that are offered by independent educators, such as Birthworks or Bradley classes, as opposed to those offered through the hospital. It is best to join a class that includes couples planning on giving birth at home, even if the woman plans to deliver in a birth center or hospital. This is to insure that the information given is not slanted for the purpose of making her into a compliant hospital patient, but that it is meant to empower and educate her about her choices.

- Plan on giving birth as naturally as possible. One medical intervention tends to lead to another, and then another. Each brings along with it many negative side effects and potential dangers for her and her baby. Remember that, when unnecessary, each intervention only interferes with Nature's plan.

- Surround herself with the people, environment, and experiences that support her in connecting to her innate ability to give birth safely and naturally.

- Make sure her birth attendant knows how to support the natural birth process, as opposed to dealing with birth as a mechanical procedure fraught with danger. This knowledge is, unfortunately, not taught in medical schools.

- If she is planning to deliver at home, she should ask what her birth attendant's cesarean section or hospital transport rate is. If it is more than 10%, I suggest she find someone else to provide her care. (The current cesarean section rate in the U.S. is about 25% or more. This is completely unnecessary. In the Netherlands, where 70% of babies are born by natural childbirth attended by midwives, the cesarean section rate is about 7%. This is common in other states and countries where midwives and homebirth are the norm.)

While putting out her best effort, it is important for her to remember that each birth has a plan of its own. She can and should prepare, plan, and visualize her ideal birth, but the expectant mother must be able to surrender and let go in order to allow birth to happen. This is also true for letting go of the "ideal" birth she is wanting, and accepting the reality of the moment. Our life's lessons often come in mysterious ways.

After the birth, the new mother needs to be easy on herself and her partner, accept that she has done her best, allow for learning to occur, and take time to grieve, heal, and integrate any loses that she may have suffered. This is true whether the loss was that of the life of her child or the loss of the birth as she had wanted it. Remind her that the amount of time it takes to heal is very individual.

Remedies to Consider:

Arnica: Give a high potency dose (200c or whatever you have on hand) before a cesarean section or other difficult delivery (episiotomy, very rapid, long or traumatic birth, prolonged or difficult pushing stage, a large baby, shoulder dystocia, or forceps birth, etc.) and immediately afterwards. If you are using a 30c potency or lower, give it before the birth, and every two hours afterwards for the rest of the first day. If recovering from a cesarean section or other surgical wound, begin using *Staphysagria* 30c after the bruising and soreness has subsided (usually 1 - 2 days, or sooner if pain is the main symptom), and three to four times a day for the next week, as needed for pain. (See *Staphysagria* below.)

    Arnica will promote healing, control bleeding, prevent tearing, reduce swelling and bruising, relieve soreness, prevent shock and infections, help the uterus contract, and expel the placenta.

    It is particularly indicated when the postpartum woman feels sore and bruised in one area of her body, or all over. It is impossible, in this state, for her to find a comfortable position and she appears restless in her attempt to do so. Her chair and bed feel too hard. She does not want to be touched or approached because of the soreness. She can be irritable, wants to be left alone, and says there is nothing the matter with her when you know there is.

Bellis perennis: For bruised soreness, specifically of the abdominal wall and pelvic organs after childbirth, where *Arnica* has either not helped or has stopped helping, use *Bellis perennis*. *Bellis perennis* is particularly useful for wounds and surgery to the abdominal area. The uterus feels sore, as if squeezed. It will alleviate the bruising and soreness, prevent infections, and dramatically speed healing.

Ignatia: This is the remedy to use during an acute emotional crisis, particularly one of loss, grief, or deep disappointment. This could be after a stillbirth, the death of the newborn, placing the baby for adoption, or the birth experience not occurring as planned, i.e., such as having a cesarean instead of a vaginal birth, or a hospital birth instead of a homebirth, etc. Her expectations or ideals have clashed with reality.

The woman who will benefit from *Ignatia* either breaks down into hysterical, uncontrollable sobbing or avoids breaking down in front of others and tries to keep her feelings inside. Her frequent sighing gives away her internal turmoil. She avoids crying in front of others but cries uncontrollably when she is alone. She feels the sensation of a lump in her throat. Insomnia is a common complaint for this woman. She is often extremely self-critical and very sensitive to reprimand. Her moods are very changeable and unpredictable.

Ignatia will help to give her the inner strength to face the pain she is experiencing, to grieve her loss in a healthy manner, and to regain her inner strength. Remember to treat the other family members with *Ignatia* who may be experiencing a similar state.

Give a 30c potency 3 to 4 times a day for a few days, or as needed for grief. In an extreme crisis, give a 30c potency every 15 minutes for an hour, every hour for 3 hours, then 3 times a day for several days, or as needed.

Read more about *Ignatia* and the personal account of Bev in the chapter "Prolonged, Difficult, or Dysfunctional Labor."

Phosphorus: Will antidote the aftereffects of anesthesia if the woman feels spaced out, has a hard time coming back into her body, feels emotionally too open and vulnerable, and is anxious and fearful. One 200c dose should do it, or give a 30c three times a day for up to a few days.

Staphysagria: This remedy is specific for clean surgical wounds such as episiotomies and cesarean sections, and can be used fairly routinely after surgeries of this type. It helps these wounds to heal rapidly, minimizes pain, and prevents infections. It is to incised wounds (surgical cuts) what *Calendula* is to lacerations (irregular tears).

Use *Arnica* or *Bellis perennis* for one or two days for bruising and soreness (see *Arnica* above), and follow with *Staphysagria* 30c three times a day for up to a week. However, if pain after a cesarean is the main complaint, *Staphysagria* is the remedy to begin with. Give a 30c dose every three to four hours as needed for pain during the first day, then three times a day for a few days to one week.

Think of *Staphysagria* when a woman feels she has been violated, humiliated, assaulted, or otherwise emotionally traumatized during her labor and birth.

She feels emotionally sensitive and her physical wound is sensitive also. The anger will often be suppressed. She may feel guilt and shame instead of anger. There is disappointment and resentment about the way the birth occurred and how she was treated. There may be a history of previous incest or sexual abuse.

For information on treating injuries to the nerves or spine, perhaps after an epidural or forceps delivery, read the chapter "Injuries to the Coccyx and Spine."

CHAPTER 17

The Newborn

The transition from womb to world can be a serene and peaceful experience for the newborn. Remembering how pure, sensitive, and vulnerable she is allows you to handle the new baby with gentleness and love. Welcome the baby with low lights, soft voices, and gentle, loving touches. Place her in mother's waiting arms. Give her lots of skin to skin contact. The calming voices of mother and father are familiar to the newborn, thus comforting and reassuring her as she adjusts to the newness of the world. (Note: As already mentioned, I have chosen to use the female pronouns "she" and "her" to represent all newborns.)

It is important to keep the newborn warm and dry. Make sure the birth room is toasty warm. Gently dry off the baby with a soft cotton towel and replace it with a dry one. Also place a dry cotton cap on her head since most of the newborn's body heat is lost from the head.

Allow the cord to stop pulsating on its own before cutting it. This provides oxygen to the baby as she begins to breathe gradually on her own, allowing a smooth transition.

The newborn baby will naturally breathe on her own within the first moments of life, turning her a healthy pink color, starting from her chest area, and extending to her extremities. For those that need a bit of gentle stimulation to help them fully come into their bodies, gently drying them off is usually enough. Though the newborn needs to fully open her lungs and clear out any fluid remaining there, this will be naturally accomplished by gentle deep breathing for some, while others will cry robustly for a short while. Routine suctioning is not necessary. Simply wipe away any excess blood and fluid from the nose and mouth with a soft cloth.

A few newborns will need extra stimulation to get their breathing started. You can provide this by running your fingers gently along both sides of their spine, up and down. Be sure to remind everyone in the birth room to breathe also. It is amazing how many people at a birth hold their own breath in anticipation for the newborn!

Though most natural, unmedicated births will unfold without any complications, it is important to be prepared for the rare few where problems may occur. Babies can be born stressed from a long, difficult birth, a cord complication, shoulder dystocia, placenta complication, or some other unknown cause. There may be thick meconium which necessitates deep and thorough suctioning. A baby who lacks muscle tone and does not respond to stimulation is seriously compromised and needs emergency intervention. *The birth attendant should be trained and certified in neonatal resuscitation and other emergency procedures.*

The following remedies are *not* a substitute for emergency care, but can be given along with the necessary emergency measures and/or while waiting for emergency transport to the nearest hospital.

The dose for a newborn is the same as for an adult. To prevent possible gagging or spitting out of the remedy, crush a dose between 2 spoons and place the resulting powder into the baby's mouth. You can also dissolve the remedy in water, which is especially convenient if you need to give a frequently repeated dose. Add one pellet or tablet to about 4 ounces of water, stir vigorously 15 - 20 times, and place a small amount in the baby's mouth. The remedy does not need to be dissolved before giving a dose. Stir vigorously again before each dose. Cover the cup with a clean piece of paper between doses.

In critical situations, such as neonatal asphyxia, use a 200c potency, or the highest potency you have on hand. The response should be almost immediate with the right remedy. Repeat the remedy up to every 10 seconds and change it if there is no response after 2 doses. Then repeat only as needed, if symptoms should begin to return.

First Remedy to Consider:

Arnica: The first remedy to consider after a traumatic birth, especially with any injury to the soft tissue such as bruising or cephalhematoma (a swelling containing blood on the head of the baby). The injury may have been from a variety of causes including long labor and second stage, large baby (in proportion to the size of the mother's pelvis), forceps delivery, vacuum extraction, scalp electrode, or breech birth. (Note: Second stage is from the time of full dilation of the cervix until the baby is born. This is when the mother is actively pushing.) *Arnica* will help to reabsorb the blood, reduce the swelling, and also heal any physical-emotional shock that may be there. Emotional shock, without any physical injury, will also respond well to a dose of *Arnica*.

For asphyxia, especially after an instrument delivery or other traumatic birth, where the baby has been injured, particularly with bruising or cephalhematoma, give *Arnica*. It will reactivate the baby's stunned reflexes.

If the nursing mother is taking it also, it will pass through to her breastmilk and the baby will get a dose simultaneously. However, with clear indications for the baby, give it orally to the newborn as well.

Rachelle's baby girl was born after a fairly rapid 5 hour labor, including 15 minutes of second stage. Her newborn's breathing was shallow and labored. She responded minimally to tactile stimulation. Her eyes remained shut, though the lights were very low in the room, and her muscle tone was moderate. The baby seemed to not be fully in her body. I put one pellet of *Arnica* 200c in some water, stirred, and placed a small amount of this liquid in her mouth with the teaspoon. Immediately, her eyes opened and she looked intently into mine. Her breathing deepened and became more regular. She was ready to nurse at her mother's breast.

Other Remedies to Consider:

Aconite: This remedy will quickly calm an extremely frightened newborn. Use it for birth trauma where the baby is very distressed and frightened. This can be from the birth itself (traumatic, very long or very short labor) or from vicarious fears experienced by the mother during pregnancy or labor. Think of it if there has been physical abuse during the pregnancy or other frightening experiences.

Use *Aconite* for asphyxia from extreme fear (see *Opium*). The eyes, in this case, will usually appear wide open and staring. The baby may be limp, purplish, or pale in color, with shallow breathing, or will make no attempt to breathe, has a slow, weak, or imperceptible pulse, and hot and dry skin. *Aconite* is also effective for treating retention of urine in an otherwise normal newborn after a severe fright.

Antimonium tartaricum: For respiratory distress from fluid in the respiratory tract. The baby's throat and lungs are full of mucus, which you will hear rattling. The respiration rate is accelerated. This is the main remedy for meconium aspiration with the above symptoms. In extreme cases there will be severe rattling, gasping, breathlessness, paleness, especially of the face, and imminent death.

Camphora is the remedy to use if *Antimonium tartaricum* seems indicated but fails to act.

Arnica: See above under "First Remedy to Consider."

Arsenicum album: Richard Moskowitz, M.D., finds this, in his experience, to be the best remedy for severely depressed babies who are limp, pale, appear lifeless, and who show little or no respiratory effort. He suggests its use when there are no other distinctive symptoms that would indicate another remedy.

Belladonna: Recommended for neonatal asphyxia when the baby lies motionless, with staring, bloodshot eyes, red face, dilated pupils, jerking and twitching of muscles, and hot, moist skin.

Camphora: Similar to *Antimonium tartaricum*. It is useful following meconium aspiration, and should be used when *Antimonium tartaricum* fails to act.

Camphora is useful if baby is close to death. The pulse is small and weak. The body and limbs are icy cold and blue (*Antimonium tartaricum* is characteristically pale).

Carbo vegetabilis: To improve oxygenation of the newborn. Classically, *Carbo vegetabilis* has been used for asphyxia where the baby appears near death. These babies appear collapsed, limp, flaccid, cold, and do not react to stimulation. The whole body is white, heart sounds are hardly audible, and the pulse is intermittent and thready. This remedy is known as a "corpse reviver." (See *Arsenicum album*.)

Richard Moskowitz, M.D., finds *Carbo vegetabilis* especially useful, however, when the baby is mildly or moderately depressed, deeply or persistently cyanotic, and slow to respond, but making some efforts to breathe. He uses it for respiratory distress and persistent cyanosis from a tightly wrapped cord (see *Laurocerasus*).

Carbo vegetabilis is a great replacement for the oxygen tank when improvement of the fetal heart rate is needed. This often occurs during the pushing stage, and a dose of *Carbo vegetabilis* given to the mother will bring the baby's heartbeat back up.

China: Use *China* for neonatal asphyxia and unconsciousness after a great loss of blood by the mother during labor.

Digitalis: A rarely needed remedy for respiratory distress of babies born with congestive heart failure or congenital heart disease. It acts as a cardiac stimulant. A very slow pulse is the chief characteristic. The baby's pulse is weak, abnormally slow, and irregular. Any movement increases the rapidity of the pulse, but causes no increase in the force of the heart's beat. The child is much worse from any motion or exertion. Her skin often feels icy cold despite being warmly covered.

Hypericum: For traumatic injury to the spine or nerves. Brachial palsy. For convulsions after birth due to injuries to the baby's spine. The pains shoot along the lines of nerves. There may be numbness and tingling. What *Arnica* is to the soft tissues and muscles, *Hypericum* is to the nerves and spine.

Laurocerasus: For a baby with a blue face and extremities. There may be heart valve problems or other heart abnormalities. The main remedy for strangulation from a wrapped cord. The body may exhibit a normal color or be pale, and cold. The newborn has difficulty breathing, gasps, or breathes imperceptibly. There is lack of reaction. The pulse is slow, feeble, irregular, and may be failing. There may be twitching of the muscles of the face.

These babies are better lying down and worse sitting up, which causes them to gasp. They get worse from the slightest exertion.

Opium: As I have mentioned before, this remedy is unfortunately no longer legally available in the U.S. due to the F.D.A. It is an important remedy for unconsciousness and coma, and so I have included it here. It is totally safe in homeopathic form.

Opium is indicated for asphyxia of the newborn after a severe fright (see *Aconite*). It follows *Aconite* well, if the pulse is still small and flickering, or can be used first based on its own characteristic symptoms.

Opium is similar to *Arsenicum* with the baby being pale, limp, and unresponsive. Death seems inevitable. The baby's back may be arched backwards, or the whole body is rigid. Her face may be purplish or red, and swollen. The pulse varies. Think of it if the mother was very sleepy during labor and experienced no pain where there normally would have been pain.

Rescue Remedy: *Rescue Remedy* was formulated as an emergency medicine. It is a wonderful all-purpose remedy, though not strictly homeopathic. In my experience, *Rescue Remedy* does not have the depth of action of a carefully selected homeopathic remedy, however, it is useful for its calming effect after any type of emotional or physical distress, shock, panic or fear. Use it on its own merit or if you are not sure what homeopathic remedy is indicated.

Put a few drops of the tincture in a cup of pure water. Using a teaspoon, stir, and place a small amount in the baby's mouth. It can be given once for a minor injury or distress, up to every few minutes in a serious situation, as needed.

Repertory for the Newborn

(An explanation of repertory structure and remedy grading can be found in the beginning of the "Repertory For Prolonged, Difficult, or Dysfunctional Labor," page 61. See the remedy index at the back of the book for remedy abbreviations.)

NEWBORN: *Acon., Ant-t., Arn., Ars., Bell., Camph., Carb-v., Chin., Dig., Hyper., Laur., Op.*

ASPHYXIA:
    Back arched backwards or whole body rigid: Op.
    Breathing shallow or no attempt: Acon., Ant-t., Arn., Ars., Bell., Camph., Carb-v., Chin., Laur., Op.
        If Ant-t. seems indicated but fails to act: Camph.
    Bruising, with: Arn.
    Cold, icy: Camph., Dig.
    Cyanotic: Acon., Camph., Carb-v., Chin., Dig., Laur., Op.
        Cold, icy: Camph.
        Frightened, looks and in agony: Acon.
        Heart valve problems, from, and other heart abnormalities: Laur.
        Persistently, and slow to respond: Carb-v.
        Pulse very slow, from congenital heart disease or congestive heart failure: Dig.
        Wrapped cord, from: Carb-v., Laur.
    Face red or purplish and swollen: Op.
    Face red, staring bloodshot eyes, lies motionless: Bell.
    Fear, with extreme: Acon.

ASPHYXIA (continued):
    First remedy to consider: Arn.
    Fright, after severe: Acon., Op.
        Blue all over: Acon.
        Fear, with extreme: Acon.
        Pale, limp: Acon., Op.
        Red all over: Op.
        Unresponsive: Op.
    Gasping: Ant-t., Camph., Carb-v., Laur.
        Cold, icy, blue skin: Camph.
        Heart complaints, in: Laur.
        Mucus, fluid, or meconium in respiratory
            tract, from: Ant-t.
            If Ant-t. seems indicated but fails to act:
                Camph.
        Wrapped cord, from: Carb-v., Laur.
    Heart failure, congestive, or congenital heart
        disease, born with: Dig.
    Heart valve problems and other heart
        abnormalities: Laur.
    Hot dry skin: Acon.
    Hot moist skin: Bell.
    Limp: Acon., Ars., Carb-v., Op.
        Fright, after severe: Acon., Op.
            Fear, with extreme: Acon.
            Pale, limp: Acon., Op.
                Blue all over: Acon.
                Red all over: Op.
                Unresponsive: Op.
        Severely depressed, appears lifeless: Ars.,
            Carb-v., Op.
        Mother sleepy during labor and
            experienced no pain: Op.
    Loss of blood in mother, from: Chin.
    Meconium aspiration, from: Ant-t.
        If Ant-t. seems indicated but fails to act:
            Camph.

ASPHYXIA (continued):
    Mother sleepy during labor and experienced no
        pain: Op.
    Mucus, fluid, or meconium in respiratory tract,
        from: Ant-t.
            If Ant-t. seems indicated but fails to act:
                Camph.
    Pale: Acon., Ant-t., Ars., Carb-v., Op.
    Pulse, very slow, from congenital heart disease
        or congestive heart failure: Dig.
    Purplish color: Acon.
    Respiratory rate accelerated from mucus, fluid,
        or meconium in respiratory tract: Ant-t.
            If Ant-t. seems indicated but fails to act:
                Camph.
    Respond, does not: Ars., Carb-v., Chin., Op.
        Loss of blood in mother, from: Chin.
        Mother sleepy during labor and
            experienced no pain: Op.
        Severely depressed, appears lifeless: Ars.,
            Carb-v.
    Severely depressed, appears lifeless: Ars.,
        Carb-v.
    Skin hot and moist: Bell.
    Traumatic birth, after: Acon., Arn.
        Bruising, with: Arn.
        Fear, with extreme: Acon.
    Wrapped cord, from: Carb-v., Laur.

BRACHIAL PALSY: Hyper.

BRUISING: Arn.

CEPHALHEMATOMA: Arn.

FEAR, EXTREME, to help calm: Acon.

FETAL HEART RATE, to improve during pushing
stage: Carb-v.

FIRST REMEDY TO CONSIDER: Arn.

PULSE VERY SLOW, from congenital heart disease
or congestive heart failure: Dig.

TRAUMATIC BIRTH: Acon., Arn., Hyper.
Brachial palsy: Hyper.
Bruising, with: Arn.
Fear, with extreme: Acon.
Injury to the spine or nerves, with: Hyper.

UNCONSCIOUSNESS:
Coma: Op.
Great loss of blood in mother, from: Chin.

URINE, RETENTION OF, from extreme fear: Acon.

WRAPPED CORD, strangulation from: Carb-v.,
Laur.

Postscript

The miracle of childbirth is one of the most important passages in a woman's life. She becomes the vessel through which the physical manifestation of love occurs, the birth of a new life. Her spirit, the spirit of the child, as well as those of the others present, is awakened to the loving miracle that is life. Childbirth is meant to be a celebration of this love. With all its possible trials, tribulations, and associated pain, birth serves to affirm and strengthen the human spirit when it is approached with the dignity and reverence it merits.

Homeopathic medicine offers itself as the perfect ally in supporting this birth process. Its gentle, non-invasive assistance sustains the full unfoldment of nature's plan.

I sincerely hope that your knowledge of homeopathy and its many uses will mature with time and that this book has helped in that aspiration. I welcome your comments, insights, and sharing of experiences.

Betty Idarius
P.O. Box 388
Talmage, CA 95481
(707) 463-3739
E-mail: bidarius@saber.net

Resources

Homeopathic References:

- Brennan, Patty, *Guide to Homeopathic Remedies for the Birth Bag*. Ann Arbor, Michigan: Trusting Nature, 1997.

- Castro, Miranda, *Homeopathy for Pregnancy, Birth, and Your Baby's First Year*. New York, New York: St. Martin's Press, 1993. Highly recommended.

- Coppe Mouscron, Yves, Dr., *Pregnancy, Parturition, Homoeopathy*. Belgium: Homeoden Bookservice.

- Farrington, Harvey, M.D., "Homeopathy in the New-Born Infant." Journal Of The American Institute Of Homeopathy, May, 1955.

- Guernsey, Henry, M.D., *The Application of the Principles and Practice of Homeopathy to Obstetrics*. New Delhi, India: B. Jain Publishers, 1990.

- Hahnemann, Samuel, *Organon of the Medical Art*. Edited by Wenda Brewster O'Reilly. Redmond, Washington: Birdcage Books, 1996.

- Jansen, Jan, *Synthetic Bedside Repertory for Gestation, Childbirth and Childbed*. The Netherlands: Merlijn Publishers, 1992.

- Morrison, Roger, *Desktop Guide to Keynotes and Confirmatory Symptoms*. Albany, California: Hahnemann Clinic Publishing, 1993.

- Moskowitz, Richard, *Homeopathic Medicines for Pregnancy and Childbirth.* Berkeley, California: North Atlantic Books, 1992. Highly recommended.

- Shiloh, Jana, *Homeopathy for Birthing.* Sedona, Arizona: Rocky Mountain Homeopathics, 1990.

- Shiloh, Jana, "Homeopathic Remedies for Labor and Birth." Mothering, Summer 1990.

- Touw, Rob van der and Wilmshurst, John, *The Homeopathic Guide to Obstetrics.* Compiled mainly from lectures, seminar notes, and tapes of Ananda Zaren.

- Vermeulen, Frans, *Concordant Materia Medica, 2nd edition.* The Netherlands: Merlijn Publishers, 1997.

- Warkentin, David Kent, *MacRepertory and Referenceworks.* San Rafael, California: Kent Homeopathic Associates.

- Wells, Henrietta, *Homeopathy for Children.* Rockport, Massachusetts: Element, Inc., 1993.

- Yasgur, Jay, *A Dictionary of Homeopathic Medical Terminology, 4th edition.* Greenville, Pennsylvania: Van Hoy Publishers, 1998.

- Yingling, W. A., *The Accoucher's Emergency Manual.* New Delhi, India: B. Jain Publishers, 1988.

Childbirth References:

- Arms, Suzanne, *Birthing the Future (Immaculate*

Deception II: A Fresh Look at Childbirth). Berkeley, California: Celestial Arts, 1994 and 1996.

- Baldwin, Rahima, *Special Delivery*. Berkeley, California: Celestial Arts, 1986.

- Cohen, Nancy Wainer & Estner, Lois J., *Silent Knife: Cesarean Prevention & Vaginal Birth After Cesarean*. South Handley, Massachusetts: Bergin & Garvey Publishers, Inc., 1983.

- Davis, Elizabeth, *Heart and Hands*. Berkeley, California: Celestial Arts, 1997.

- Frye, Anne, *Healing Passage, A Midwife's Guide to the Care and Repair of the Tissues Involved in Birth, 5th edition*. Portland, Oregon: Labrys Press, 1995.

- Frye, Anne, *Understanding Diagnostic Tests in the Childbearing Year, 6th edition*. Portland, Oregon: Labrys Press, 1997.

- Gascoigne, Stephen, *The Manual of Conventional Medicine for Alternative Practitioners*. Great Britain: Jigme Press, 1993.

- Gaskin, Ina May, *Spiritual Midwifery, 3rd edition*. Summertown, Tennessee: The Book Publishing Company, 1990.

- International Childbirth Education Association, Inc., "ICEA Position Paper: Epidural Anesthesia for Labor." November, 1987. ICEA, P.O. Box 20048, Minneapolis, Minnesota, 55420.

- Kitzinger, Sheila, *The Complete Book of Pregnancy and Childbirth*. New York, New York: Alfred A. Knopf, 1997.

- Klaus, Marshall H., M.D., and Phyllis H., *The Amazing Newborn: Making the Most of the First Weeks of Life.* Redding, Massachusetts: Perseus Books, 1998.

- Varney, Helen, C.N.M., M.S.N., *Varney's Midwifery, Third Edition.* Sudbury, Massachusetts: Jones and Bartlett Publishers, 1997.

Self-Care Homeopathic Books:

- Castro, Miranda, *The Complete Homeopathy Handbook.* N.Y., N.Y.: St. Martin's Press, 1991.

- Cummings, Stephen and Ullman, Dana, *Everybody's Guide to Homeopathic Medicines.* New York, New York: Tarcher-Putnam, 1997.

- Panos, Maesimund M.D., *Homeopathic Medicine at Home.* Los Angeles, California: Jeremy P. Tarcher, Inc., 1980.

- Reichenberg-Ullman, Judyth and Ullman, Robert, *Homeopathic Self-Care.* Rocklin, California: Prima Publishing, 1997.

Sources Of Homeopathic and Childbirth Books:

- Birth & Life Bookstore, 141 Commercial St. N.E., Salem, Oregon 97301, (800) 443-9942 or (503) 371-4445. E-mail: onecascade@worldnet.att.net. Website: www.1cascade.com.

- Minimum Price, P.O. Box 2187, Blaine, Washington 98231, (800) 663-8272 or (604) 597-4757. E-mail: orders@minimum.com. Website: www.minimum.com.

- Homeopathic Educational Services, 2124 Kittredge Street, Berkeley, California 94704, (800) 359-9051 or (510) 649-0294. E-mail: mail@homeopathic.com. Website: www.homeopathic.com.

Homeopathic Pharmacies:

- Boericke and Tafel, 2381 Circadian Way, Santa Rosa, California 95407, (800) 876-9505 or (707) 571-8232. E-mail: bandt@boericke.com

- Boiron, 6 Campus Blvd., Bldg. A, Newtown Square, Pennsylvania 19073 and 98C West Cochran Street, Simi Valley, California 93065, (800) 258-8823 or (805) 582-9091. E-mail: cbs@boiron.fr. Website: www.boiron.fr.

- Dolisos, 3014 Rigel Avenue, Las Vegas, Nevada 89102, (800) 365-4767 or (702) 871-7153. Sells a reasonably priced 48 remedy self-care kit.

- Hahnemann Pharmacy, 1940 4th Street, San Rafael, California 94901, (888) 427-6422 or (415) 451-6978. High quality potencies. E-mail: pharmacy@hahnemannlabs.com. Website: www.hahnemannlabs.com.

- Helios Homoeopathic Pharmacy, 97, Camden Rd., Tunbridge Wells Kent TN1 2QR, 01144-01892-536393. E-mail: pharmacy@helios.co.uk. Website: www.helios.co.uk. High quality and reasonably priced remedies.

- Standard Homeopathic, P.O. Box 61067, Los Angeles, California 90061, (800) 624-9659 or (213) 321-4284.

(Note: Not all pharmacies conform to the same high standards in preparing their high potency remedies, therefore, the quality of different potencies will vary. Low and medium potencies up to and including 30c will be of good quality from any pharmacy. For the 200c or higher potencies, ask a homeopathic practitioner in your area for a recommendation of where they obtain their remedies. I purchase my high potencies from Hahnemann Pharmacy and Helios Homoeopathic Pharmacy and can attest to the quality of all their potencies.)

Homeopathic Organizations:

- National Center for Homeopathy, 801 North Fairfax Street, Suite 306, Alexandria, Virginia 22314, (703) 548-7790. E-mail: nchinfo@igc.org. Website: www.homeopathic.org

- North American Society of Homeopaths, 1122 East Pike St., Ste. 1122, Seattle, WA 98122, (206) 720-7000. E-mail: nashinfo@aol.com. Website: www.homeopathy.org.

Midwife Organizations:

- American College of Nurse-Midwives, 818 Connecticut Ave. N.W., Suite 900, Washington, D.C., 20006, (202) 728-9860. E-mail: info@acnm.org. Website: www.midwife.org.

- International Confederation of Midwives, 10 Barley Mow Passage, Chiswick, London, England, W4 4PH, 44-181-944-6477.

- Midwives Alliance of North America (MANA), P.O. Box 175, Newton, Kansas, 67114, (888) 923-6262. E-mail: MANAinfo@aol.com. Website: www.mana.org.

Appendices

(Note: The appendices are written strictly with the pregnant woman in mind.)

Pelvic Floor (Kegel) Exercise

The pelvic floor muscles support everything inside the pelvic cavity including the uterus, bladder, and rectum. They form a figure 8 around the vagina and anus. During pregnancy and birth these muscles are particularly stressed because of the added weight they are supporting.

The good tone of the pelvic floor muscles is important to prevent urine from leaking out (if you leak a little urine when you sneeze or cough, your pelvic floor needs some serious work), to prevent constipation, and to keep the uterus from prolapsing or sliding out of the vagina. These symptoms are common in older women who have had many children without the benefit of doing pelvic floor exercises. Awareness and control of these muscles is particularly important during birth, as this allows you to release them as you push the baby out of the birth canal, thus easing birth and preventing tearing. Doing this simple exercise during pregnancy and postpartum will assure that these muscles are in good condition for the birth and will tighten up after the baby is born.

Learning to isolate the pelvic floor muscles may take some practice but is fairly straightforward. These are the muscles that contract spontaneously during lovemaking, increasing your and your partner's sensation of pleasure. The easiest way to find them is to stop your flow of urine while urinating. You can also feel them tightening around your finger if you put one finger inside your vagina. Make sure you are not contracting your thigh, stomach, or butt muscles when doing this exercise. Practice isolating only the pelvic floor muscles.

Some women will be able to contract the pelvic floor muscles for longer than others. You may find that these muscles tire and tremble easily. As with any muscle of the body, exercise makes them stronger, so be patient with yourself. With time, you will notice them becoming much stronger.

- Imagine that your pelvic floor muscles are an elevator that you are taking to the first floor, second floor, third floor, and all the way up to the top until your muscles are fully contracted. Tighten these muscles as much as you can and hold them for a count of 20. In the beginning you may find that the muscles are not strong enough and will release before you can count to 20. Just retighten and continue counting to 20 from where you left off. This constitutes one repetition. Repeat until you have done 10 repetitions. Let your muscles fully relax between repetitions to allow them to reoxygenate and to learn to release them for the birth.

Do this exercise twice a day during pregnancy and for the first six weeks postpartum. After that, do it once a day for the rest of your life. A convenient time is before getting out of bed in the morning and before going to sleep at night.

Perineal Massage

Perineal massage is a technique used to increase the possibility of delivering a baby without an episiotomy or tearing. It stretches the perineal tissues, resulting in less resistance to the birth of a baby, as the tissues make room for the delivery. Doing the massage helps you to identify those muscles and learn to relax them in response to pressure. If the muscles of the pelvic floor are relaxed, there will also be less resistance. Massaging the oil into the perineum softens the tissue, again reducing resistance.

- The massage should be done daily for at least 5 minutes, beginning about 6 weeks before your due date.

- Either you, your husband, partner, or friend can do the massage.

- A small bottle of calendula or olive oil (or your other favorite oil that is not too thick or too thin) can be used for this and then for the birth. Some women find calendula oil to be particularly effective.

- *Make yourself comfortable*, lying in a semi-seated position against some pillows.

- The first few times you do this, take a mirror and look at your perineum so you know what you are doing.

- Wash your hands with soap and water. Dip your fingers into the oil and rub it into the perineum and lower vaginal wall.

- Doing the massage: If you are doing the massage yourself, it is probably easiest to use your thumbs. Your partner can use his index fingers. Put your fingers 3 inches into the vagina and press downwards (toward the rectum) gently. Maintaining steady pressure, slide your fingers upward along the sides of the vagina, moving them in a rhythmic U or sling type movement. This move will stretch the vaginal tissue (mucosa), the muscles surrounding the vagina, and the skin of the perineum. In the beginning, you will feel tight, but with time and practice, the tissue will relax and stretch.

- Concentrate on relaxing your muscles as you apply pressure. Do *not* apply more pressure than is comfortable and that you can relax with, as this is counterproductive. Feel yourself and your perineal muscles relaxing as you massage.

- As you become comfortable with the massage, use *slightly* more pressure until the perineum just begins to sting from the tension you apply. Be very gentle and do not overdo this. You must be able to relax with the sensation. You will later recognize this stinging sensation as the baby's head is crowning and your perineum stretching around it.

- If your partner is doing the massage, you can use this time to enjoy each other's company. You may want to have relaxing music playing in the background. It is important that you communicate openly and lovingly with each other,

151

and give whatever feedback is necessary to make sure the massage is effective and enjoyable.

- You will want to communicate with your partner beforehand as to your willingness to let the massage lead into further lovemaking. This will alleviate unnecessary tension.

In addition to perineal massage, some homeopaths recommend vaginal hot packs using *Calendula* lotion to further increase the health of the perineal area and thus prevent tearing. These hot packs are wonderfully soothing when done before or after the perineal massage, but can also be done at a separate time. (Note: Read more about *Calendula* in the chapter, "Preventing and Healing a Perineal Tear or Episiotomy.")

Make a lotion by adding either 1/2 teaspoon (2 - 3 dropperfuls) of *Calendula tincture* or 2 teaspoons of *Calendula succus* or *Calendula nonalcoholic* to 8 ounces of warm water. Lotions do not keep, so make some daily as you need it. Moisten a clean washcloth with the *Calendula* lotion so that it is wet but not dripping, place the washcloth on your perineal area, cover with plastic wrap, then place a hot water bottle or heating pad on top. Do this daily for 20 minutes during the last month of pregnancy. Be sure you are lying down and comfortable. Use this time to relax, listen to calming music, speak to your baby, and positively visualize the upcoming birth.

Index

A

Aconite (Acon.) 6, 14, 40, **42-44**, 48, 53, 54, 82, **83**, 88, **131-132**, 135
acupressure 29
acupuncture 29, 33
anesthesia, antidoting the aftereffects of 126
Antimonium tartaricum (Ant-t.) 6, **132**, 133
Arnica (Arn.) 6, 15, **76**, **78**, 79, 82, **83**, **113**, 114, **116-117**, 119, **124**, 125, 126, **130-131**, 132, 134
Arsenicum (Ars.) 6, 13, 43, **44**, 56, **132**, 133, 135

B

Belladonna (Bell.) 6, 15, **44-45**, **71**, 82, **83-84**, 90, **101**, **132**
Bellis perennis (Bell-p.) 6, **78-79**, **125**, 126
Biophysical Profile 23
birth kit, assembling a 5-7
bleeding (*see* hemorrhage)
breech presentation (*see* presentation)

C

Calendula (Calen.) 6, **117-119**, 126, 152
Calendula lotion 118, 152
Camphora (Camph.) 6, 132, **133**
Cantharis (Canth.) 6, **101**
Carbo vegetabilis (Carb-v.) 6, **84**, 85, **133**
castor oil 30
Caulophyllum (Caul.) 6, 13, 14, 15, 27, 28, **38-39**, 40, 41, 42, 45, 47, 48, **71**, 82, **84**, **101**

About The Author

Betty Idarius has been working with pregnant women and their families as a midwife, counselor, and educator for over 20 years. She is licensed as a midwife in Arizona and California. Betty graduated from The Pacific Academy of Homeopathic Medicine in 1995. She has continued her study with homeopathy masters worldwide. She is currently in private practice as a classical homeopath and midwife in Ukiah, California.

Order Form

Please send me _____ copies of *The Homeopathic Childbirth Manual.*

Name: _____

Address: _____

City: _____ State: _____ Zip: _____

Country: _____ Telephone: _____

Price: $16.95 per book.   _____

Sales Tax: Add 7 1/4% sales tax for books
    shipped to a California address.   _____

Shipping and Handling:
  In the U.S.: $3.00 for one book,
    $1.00 extra for each additional book.   _____
  To Canada and Mexico: $3.00 for one book,
    $2.00 extra for each additional book.   _____
  To all other countries: Surface: $4.00 for one book,
    $2.00 extra for each additional book.
    Airmail: $8.00 for one book, $4.00 extra for each
    additional book.   _____

Allow 30 days delivery in the U.S., Canada, or Mexico; 60 days delivery to all other countries (unless shipped airmail).

TOTAL ENCLOSED: _____

Mail order form and check or money order to:

Idarius Press
P.O. Box 388
Talmage, CA 95481
(707) 463-3739
E-mail: bidarius@saber.net
Website: www.saber.net/~bidarius